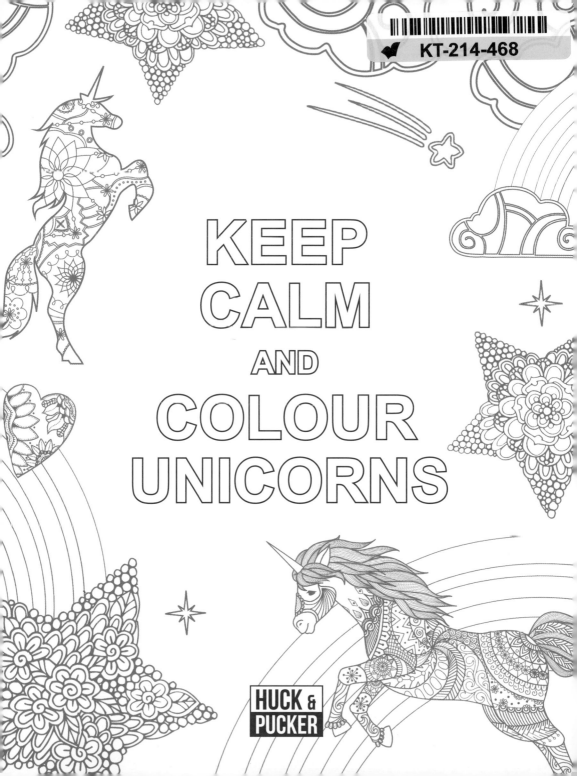

KEEP CALM AND COLOUR UNICORNS

HUCK & PUCKER

At the end of your brush is
the tip of your soul.

Andrew Hamilton

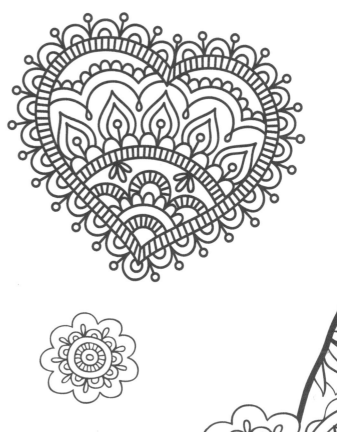

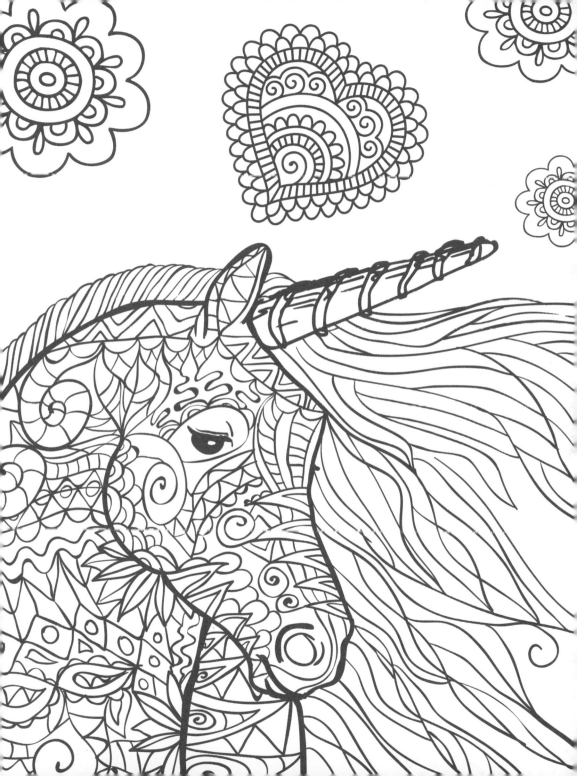

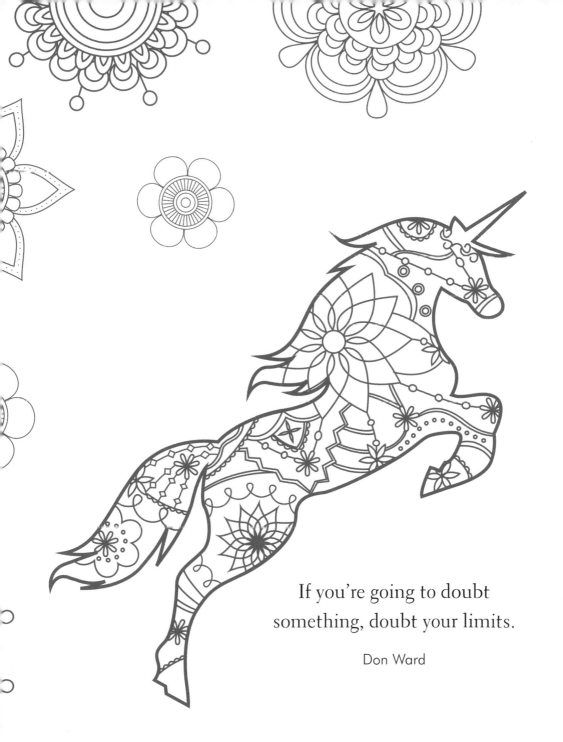

If you're going to doubt
something, doubt your limits.

Don Ward

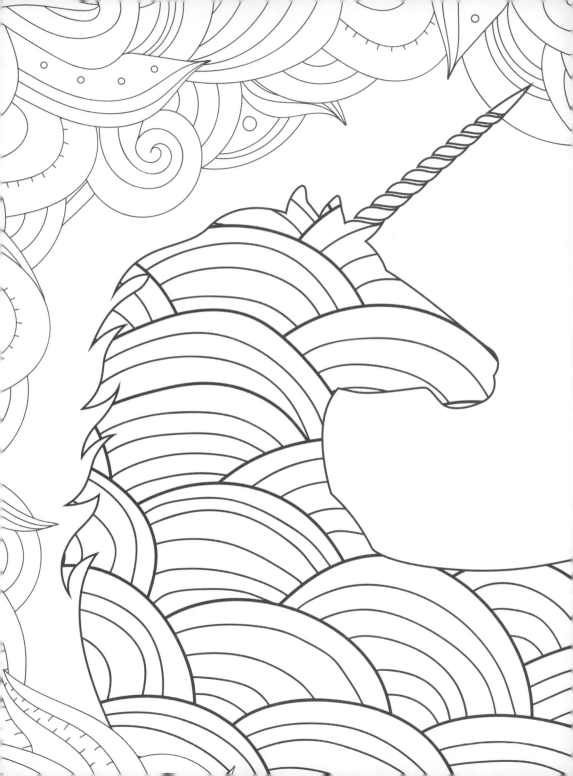

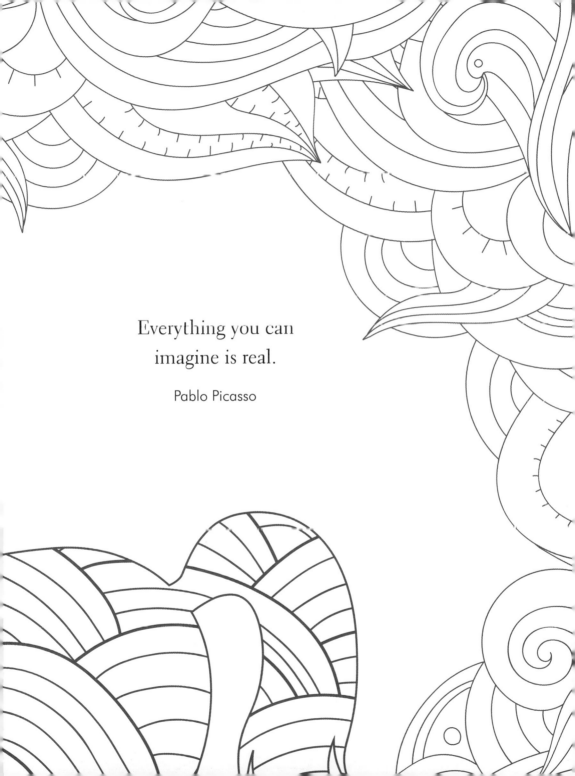

Everything you can
imagine is real.

Pablo Picasso

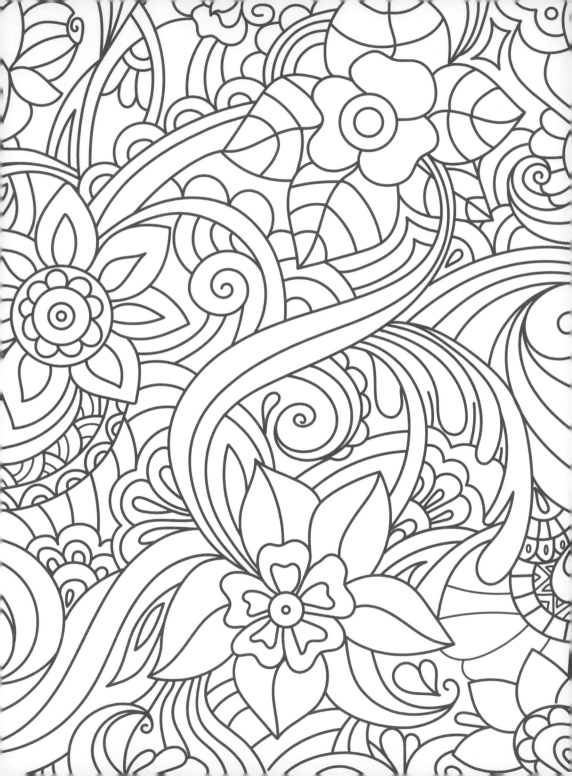

Creativity involves breaking out
of established patterns in order to
look at things in a different way.

Edward de Bono

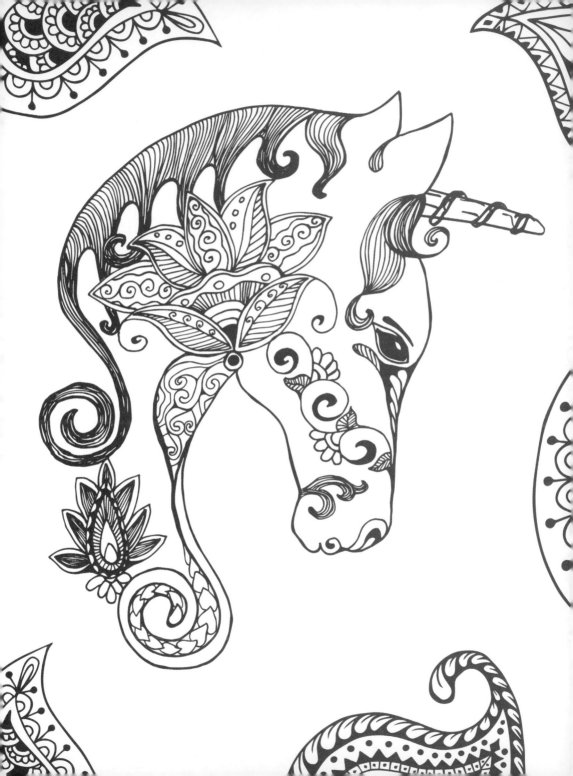

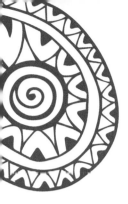
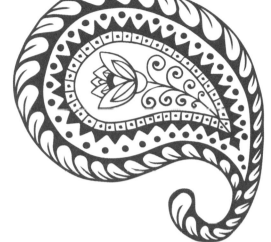

What we do flows
from who we are.

Paul Vitale

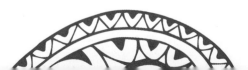

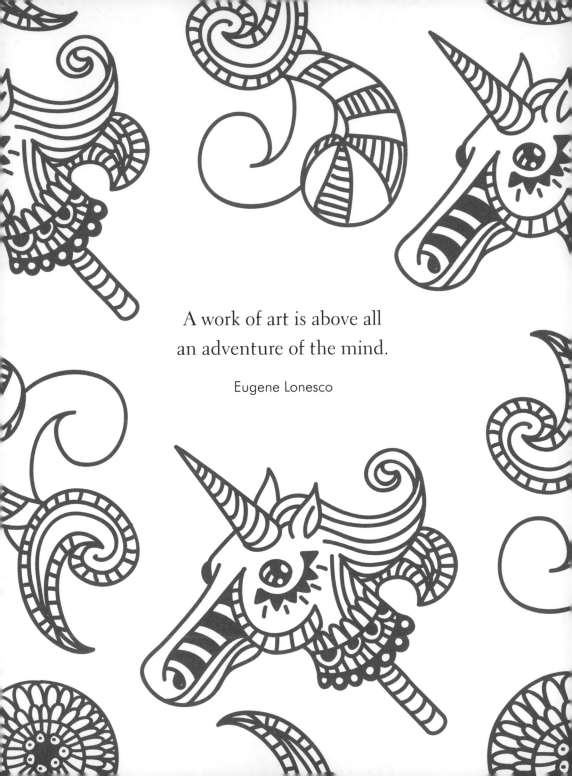

A work of art is above all
an adventure of the mind.

Eugene Ionesco

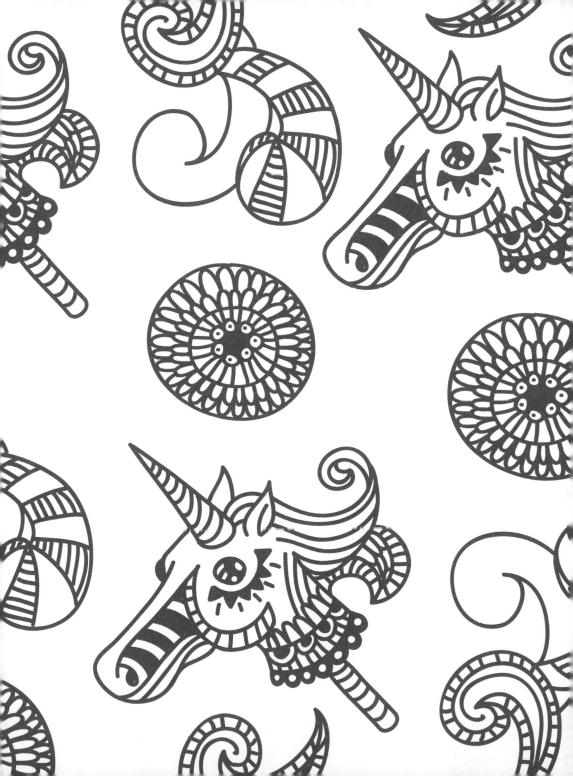

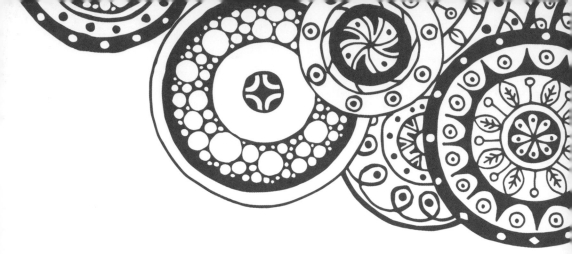

Energy and persistence
conquer all things.

Benjamin Franklin

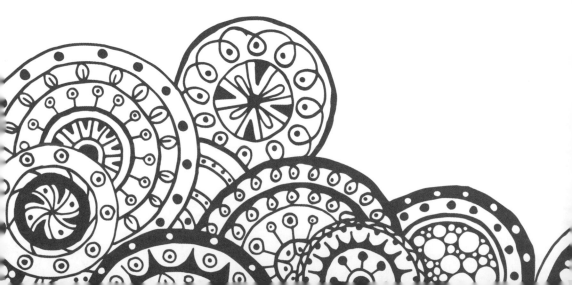

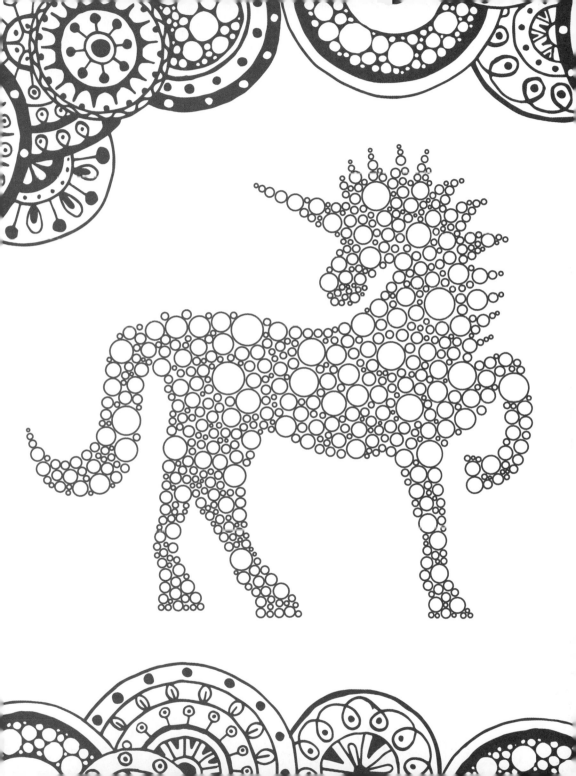

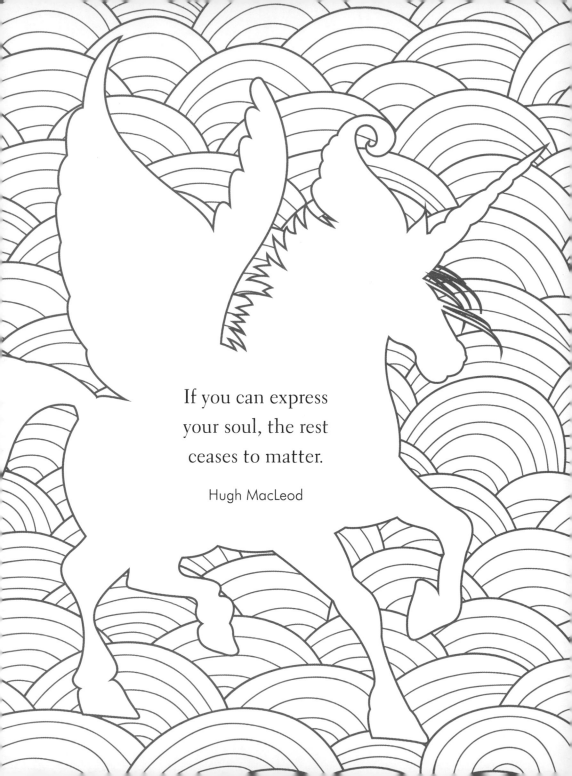

If you can express
your soul, the rest
ceases to matter.

Hugh MacLeod

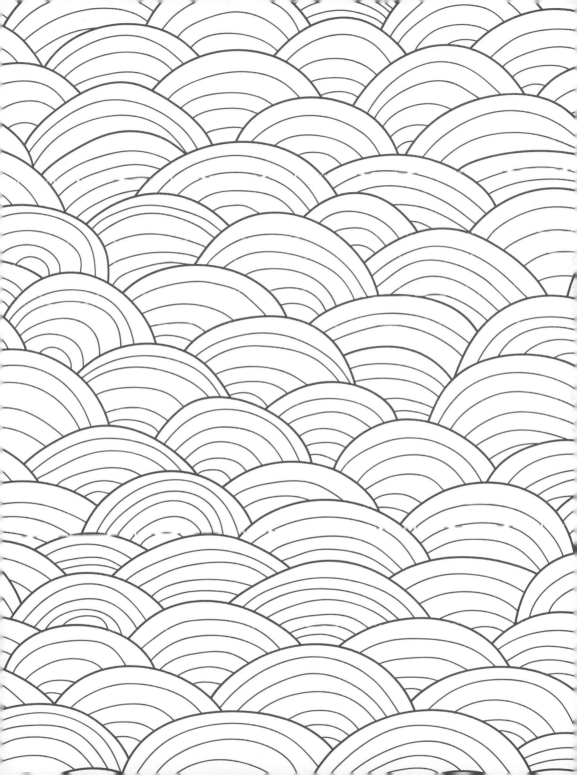

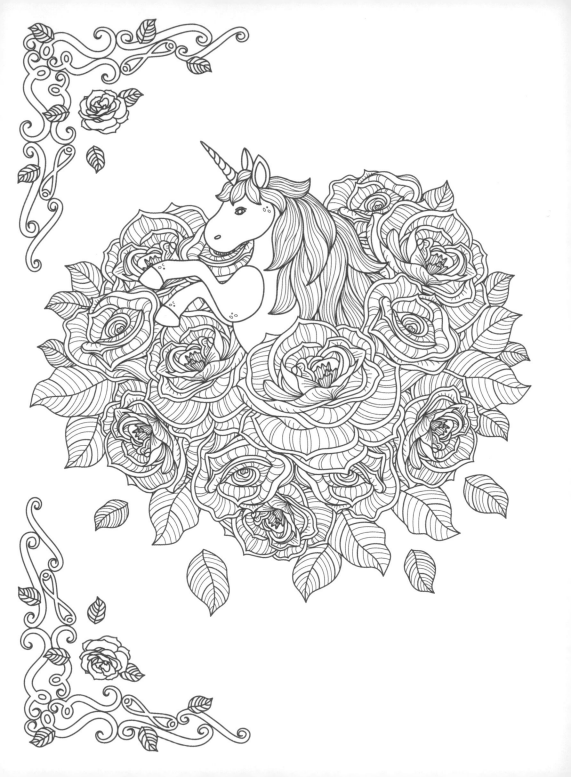

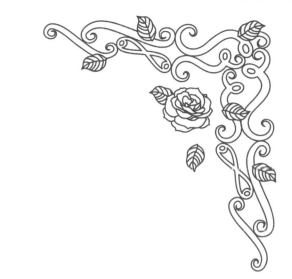

Wheresoever you go,
go with all your heart.

Confucius

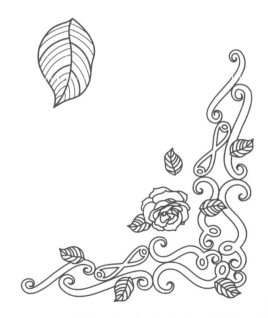

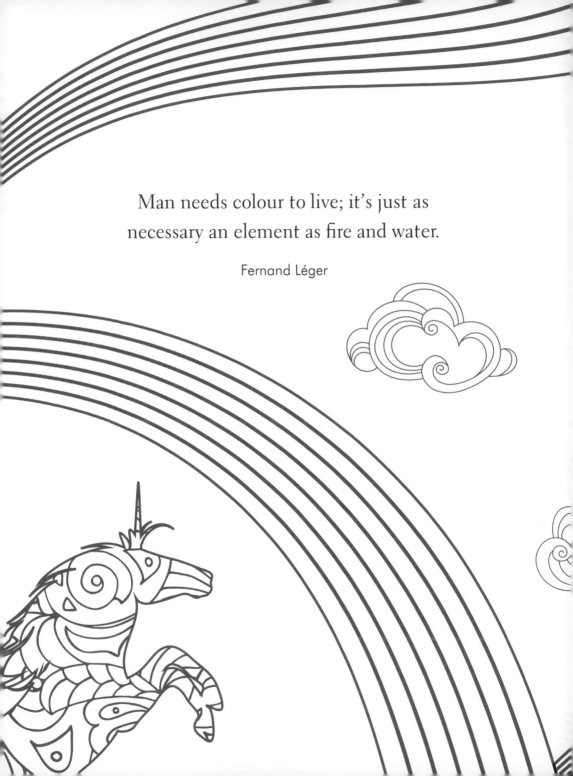

Man needs colour to live; it's just as necessary an element as fire and water.

Fernand Léger

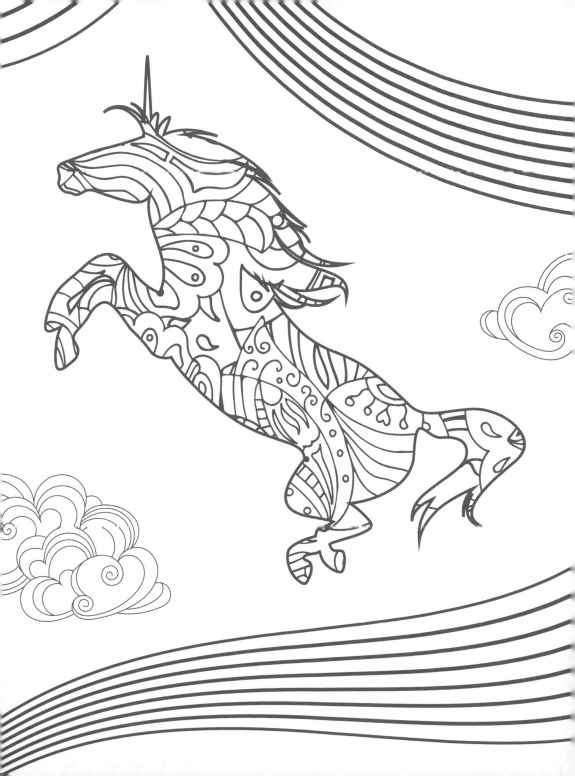

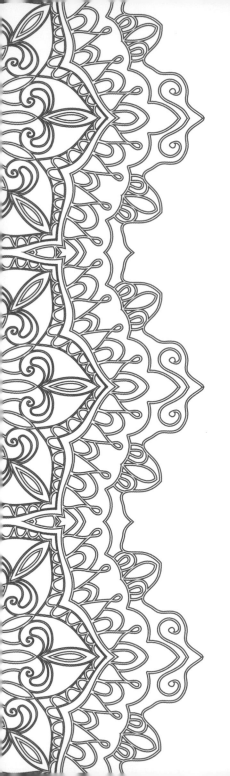

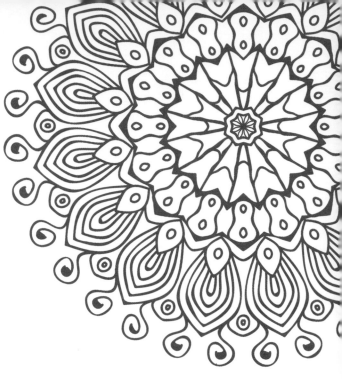

Don't let them tame you.

Isadora Duncan

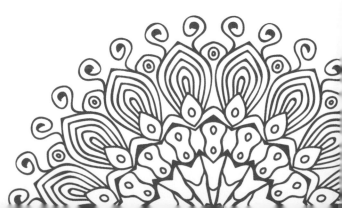

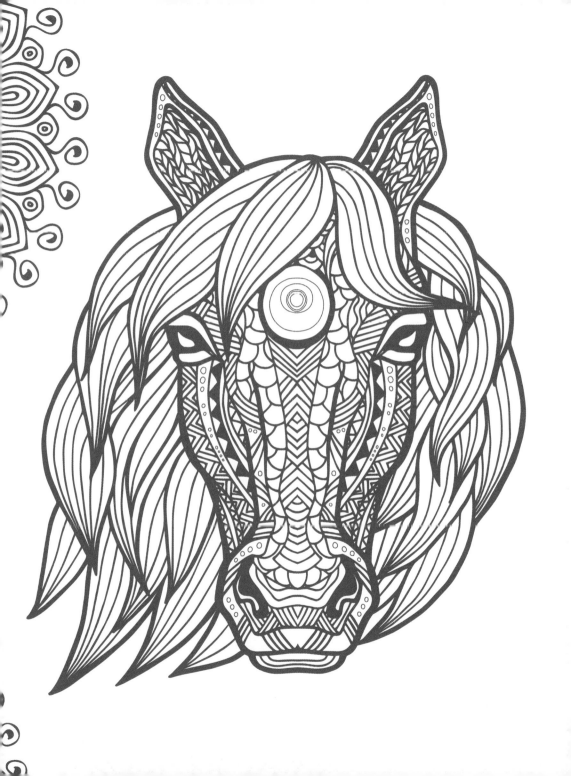

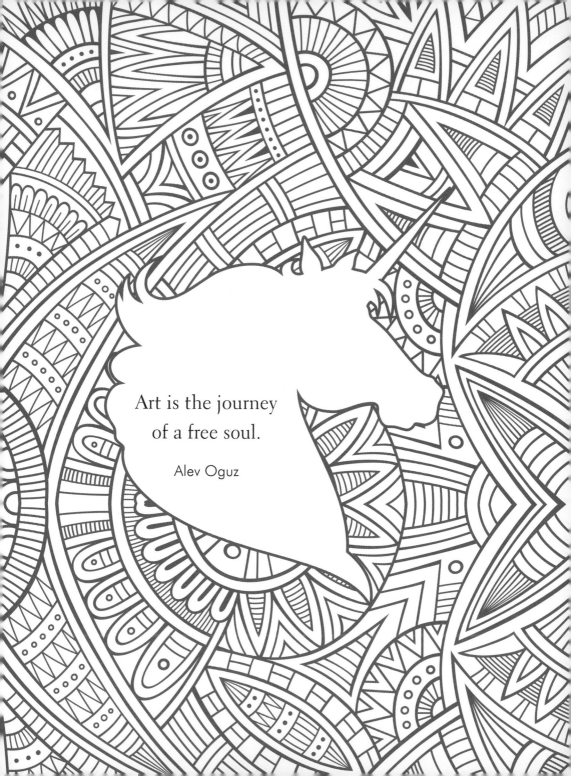

Art is the journey
of a free soul.

Alev Oguz

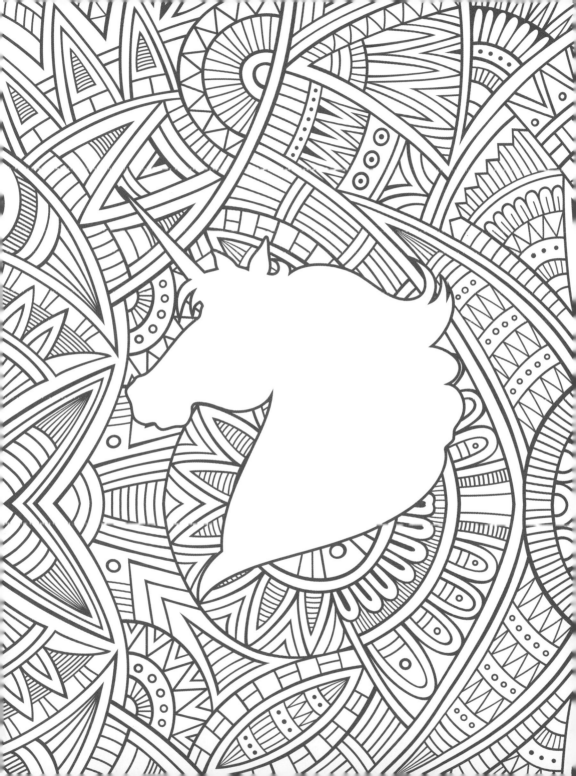

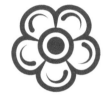

Expand your dreams…
dare to tap into your greatness.

Robin Sharma

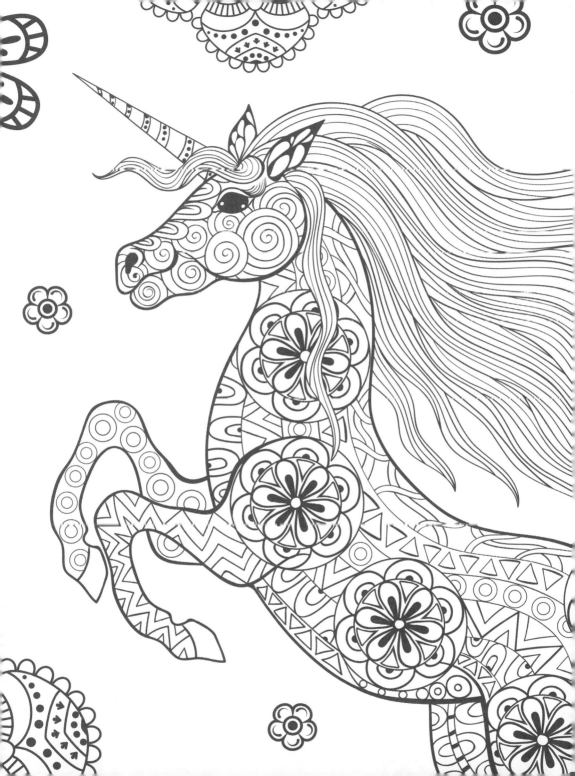

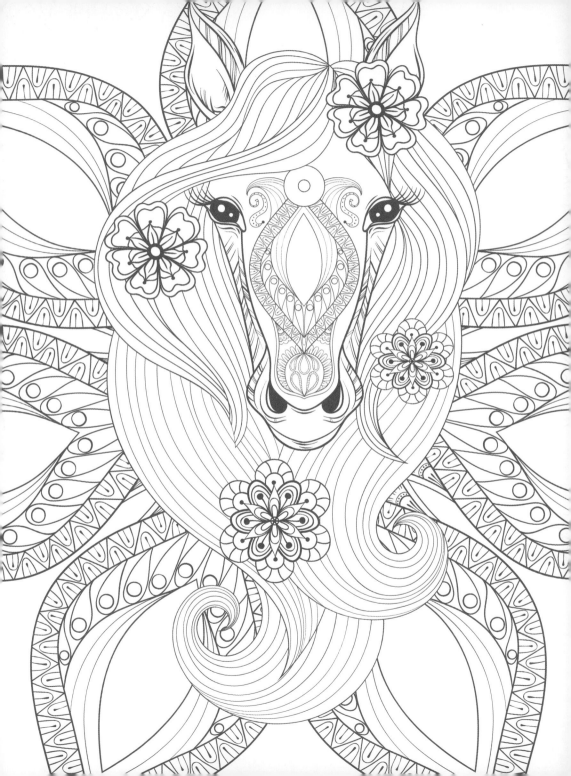

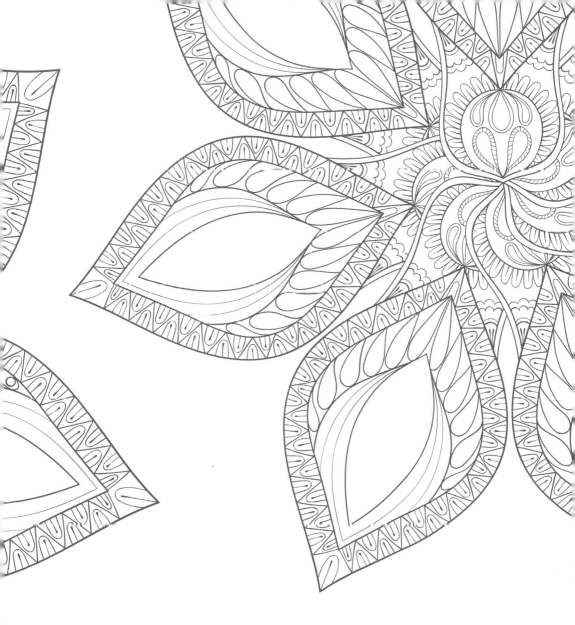

Colour is a power which
directly influences the soul.

Wassily Kandinsky

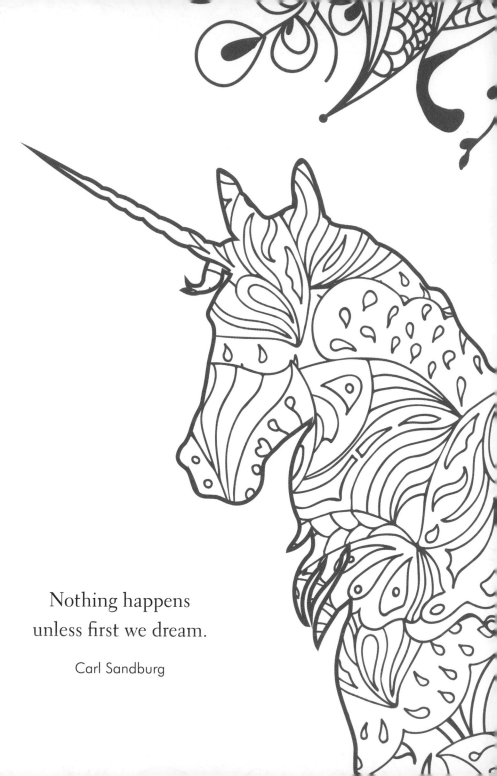

Nothing happens
unless first we dream.

Carl Sandburg

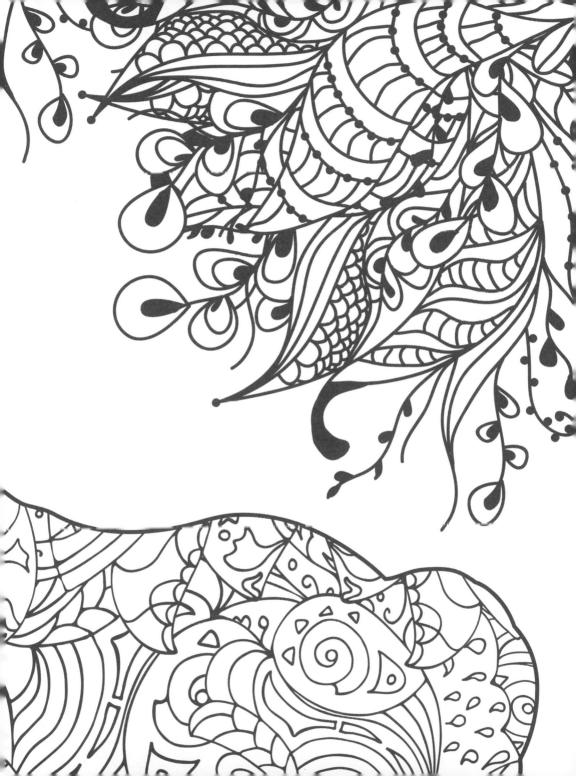

Red is passion-lit,
orange is flowerageous,
yellow is suntastic,
pink is lipsensual,
green is lifebursting,
blue is skyful, purple
is berrydancing.

Terri Guillemets

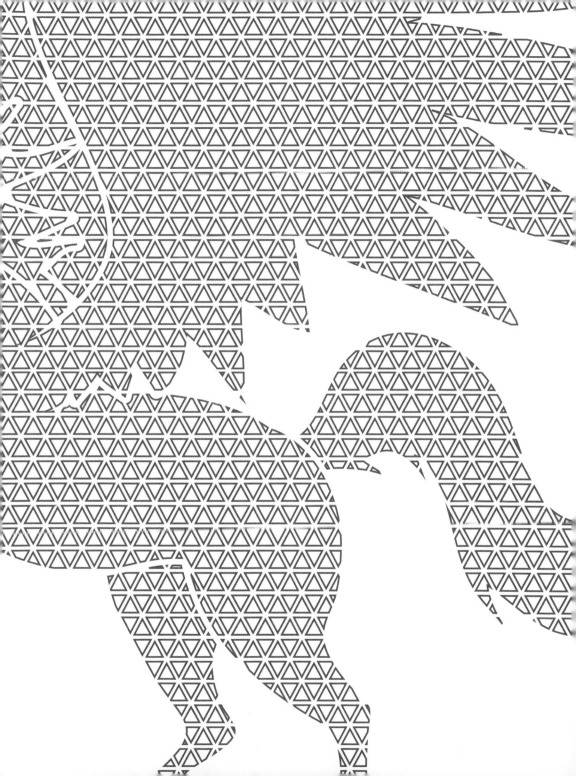

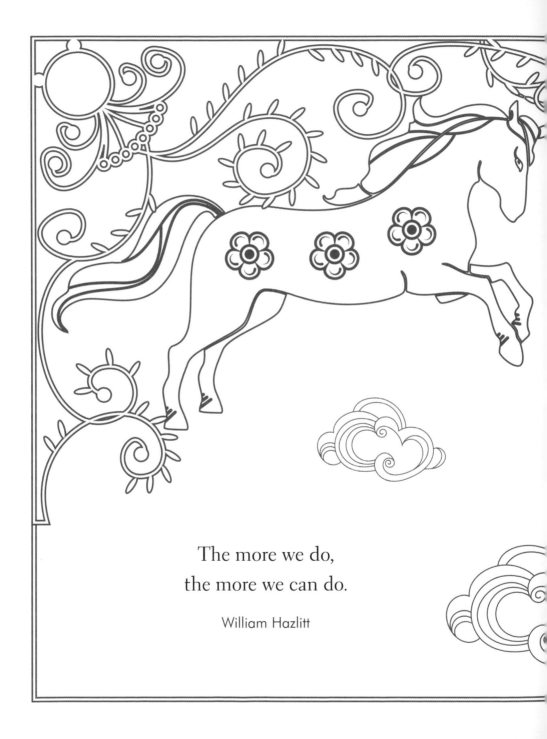

The more we do,
the more we can do.

William Hazlitt

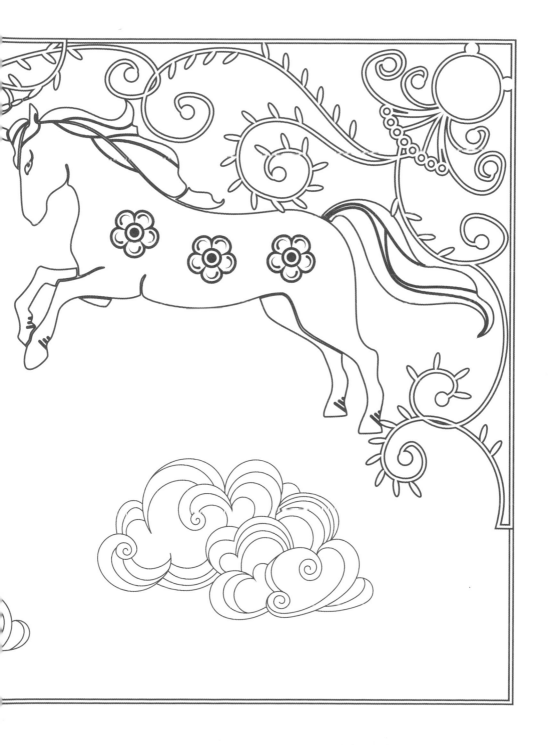

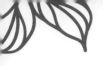

Be brave enough to live life creatively.
The creative is the place where
no one else has ever been.

Alan Alda

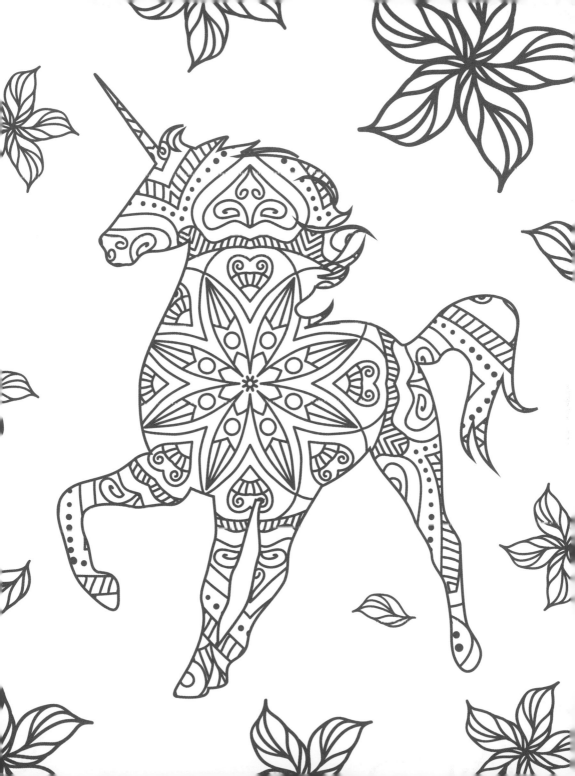

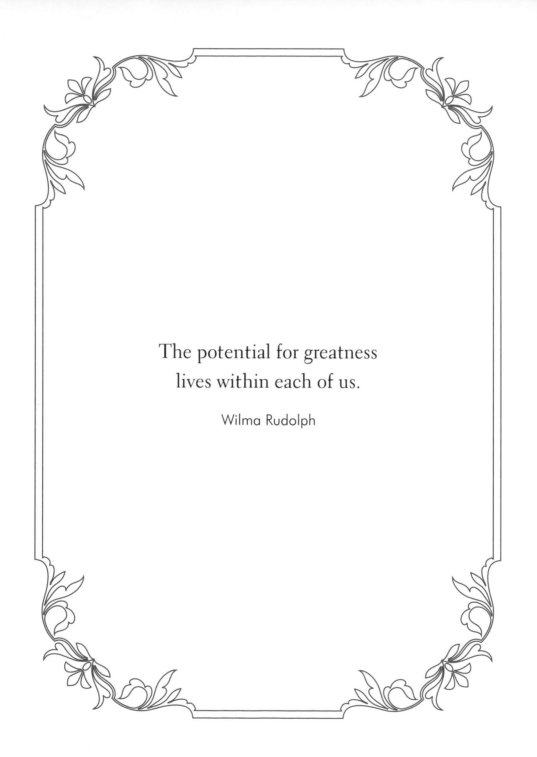

The potential for greatness
lives within each of us.

Wilma Rudolph

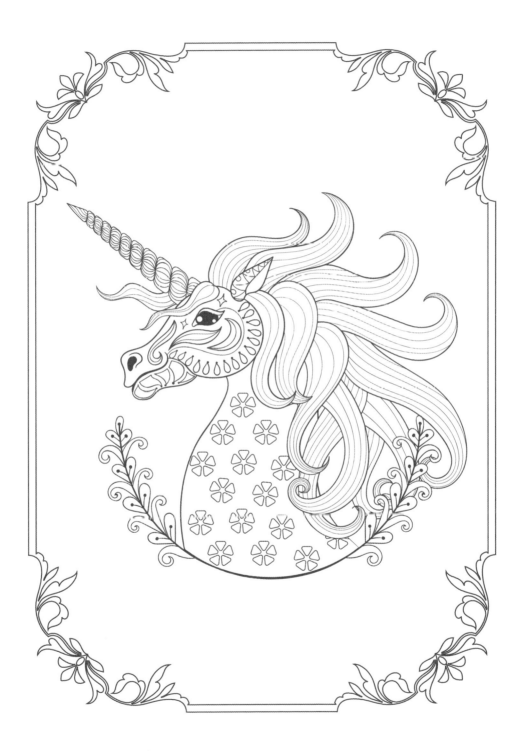

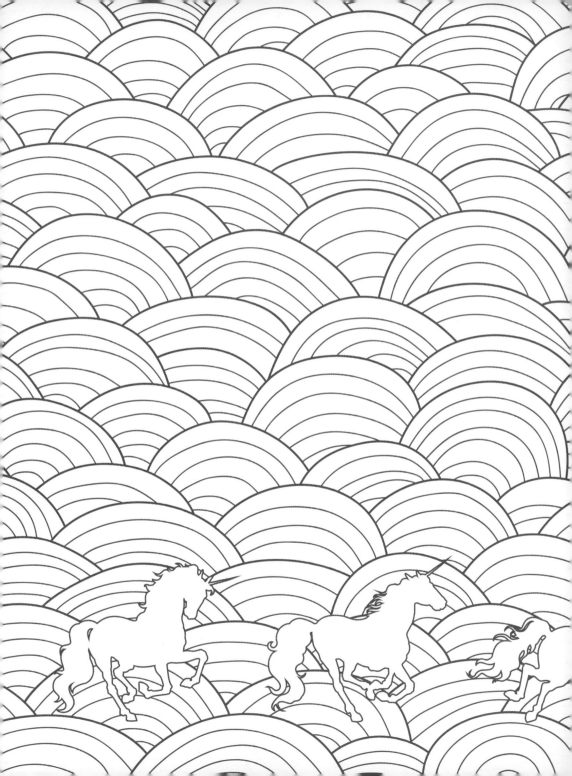

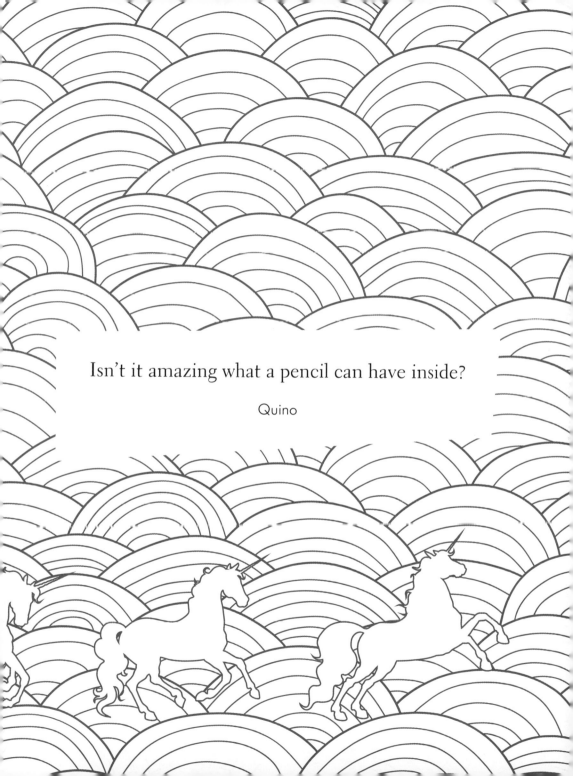

Isn't it amazing what a pencil can have inside?

Quino

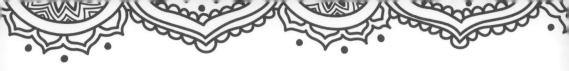

There is just one life
for each of us: our own.

Euripides

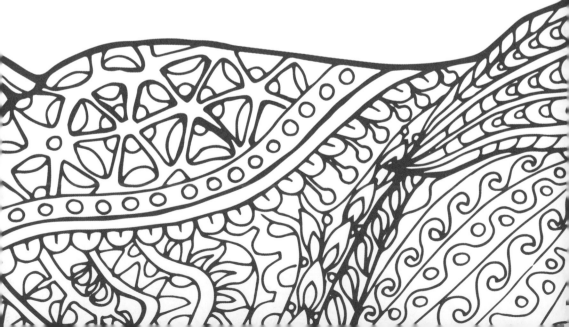

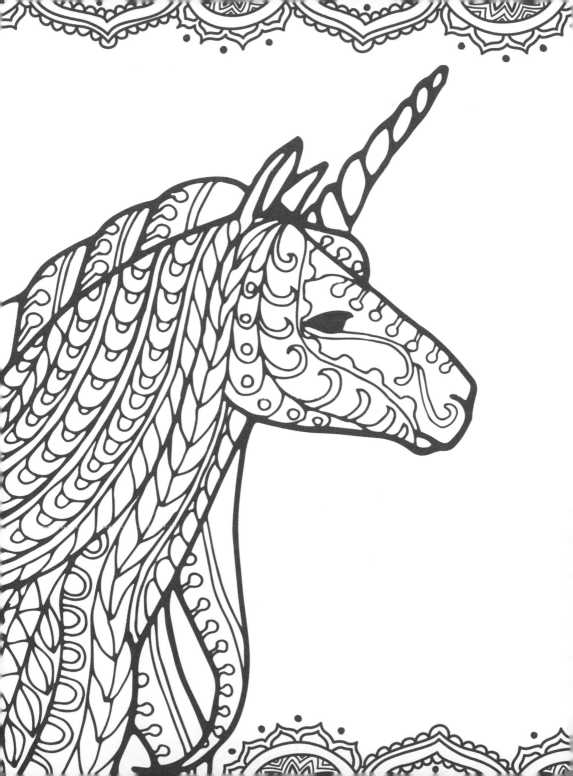

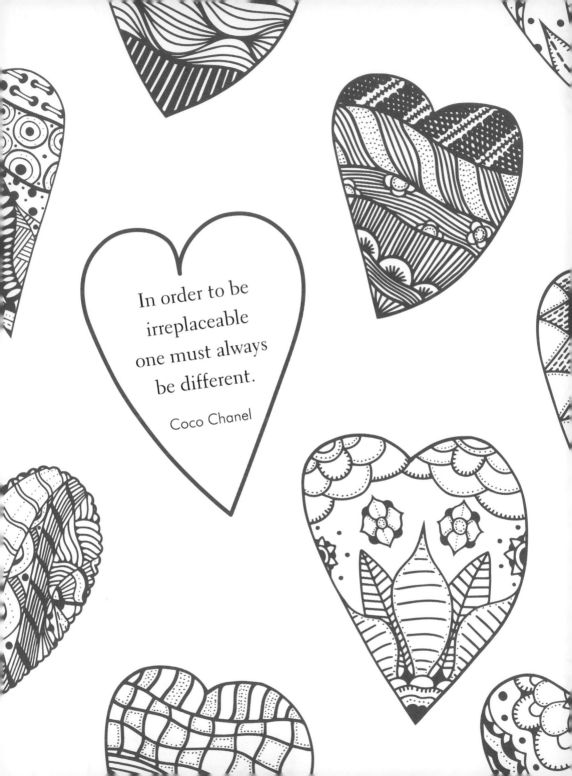

In order to be
irreplaceable
one must always
be different.

Coco Chanel

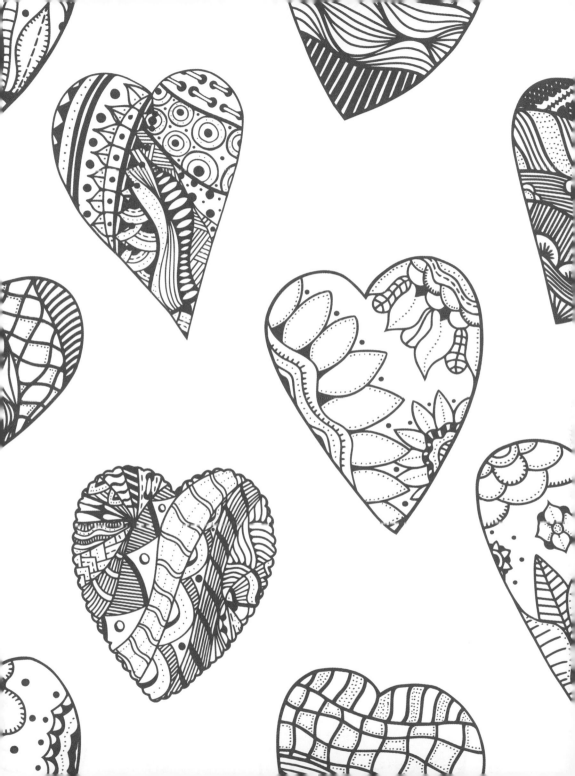

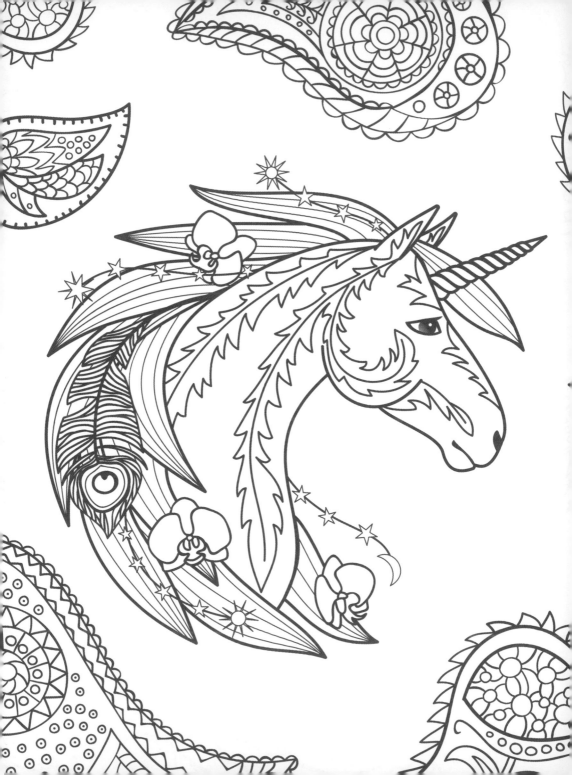

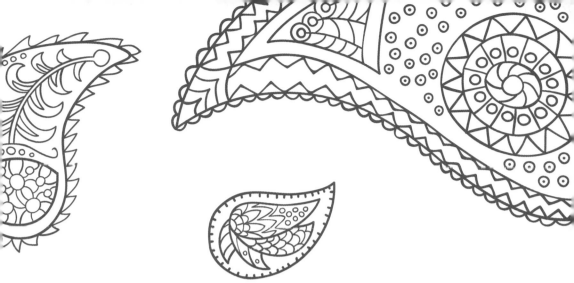

Know and believe in yourself, and what
others think won't disturb you.

William Feather

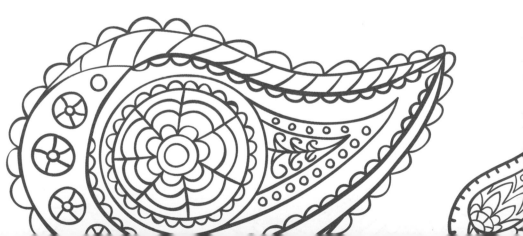

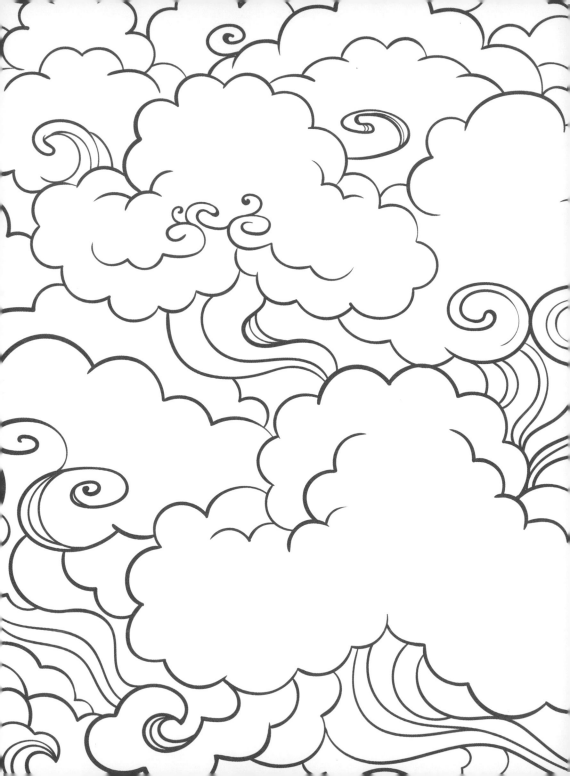

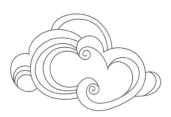

To draw, you must close your eyes and sing.

Pablo Picasso

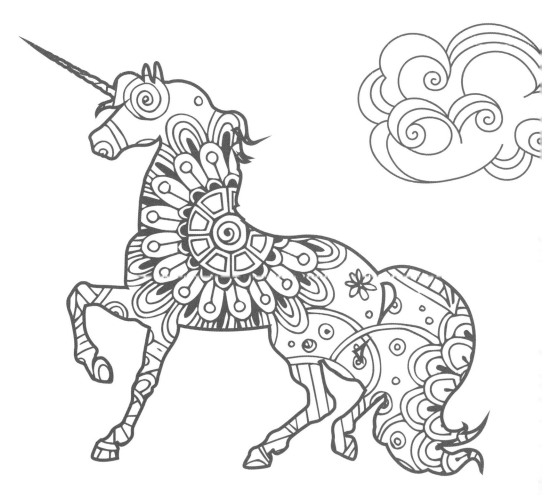

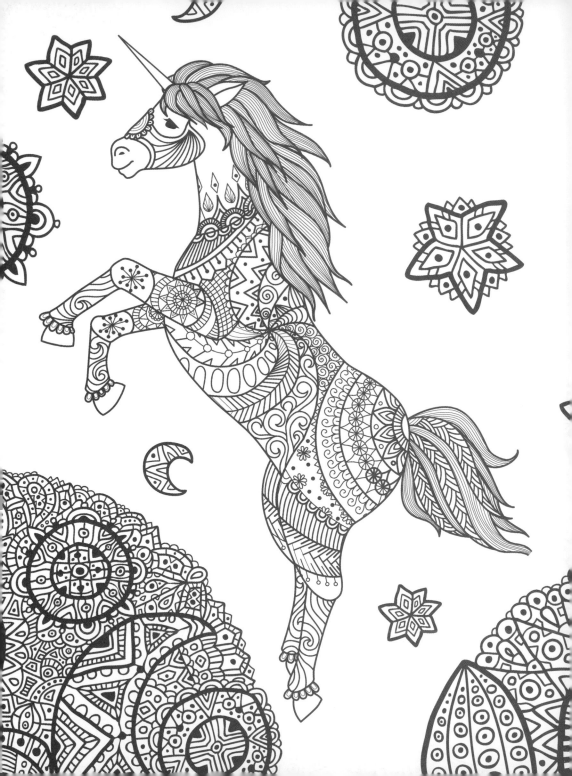

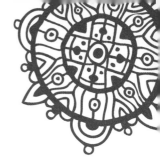

Let perseverance be your engine
and hope be your fuel.

H. Jackson Brown Jr

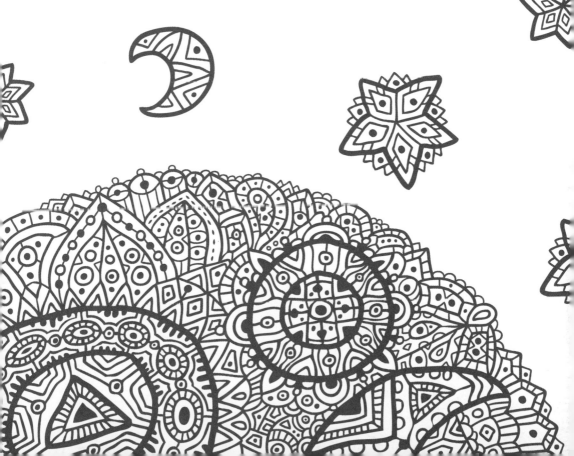

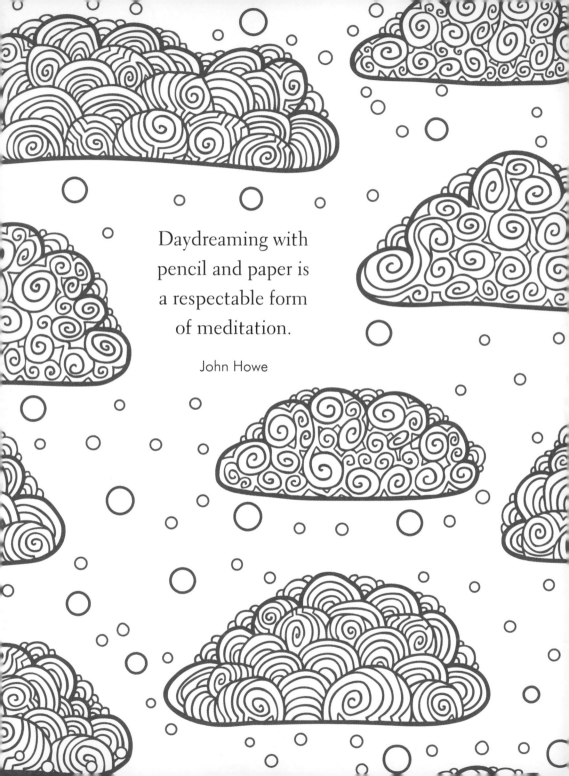

Daydreaming with
pencil and paper is
a respectable form
of meditation.

John Howe

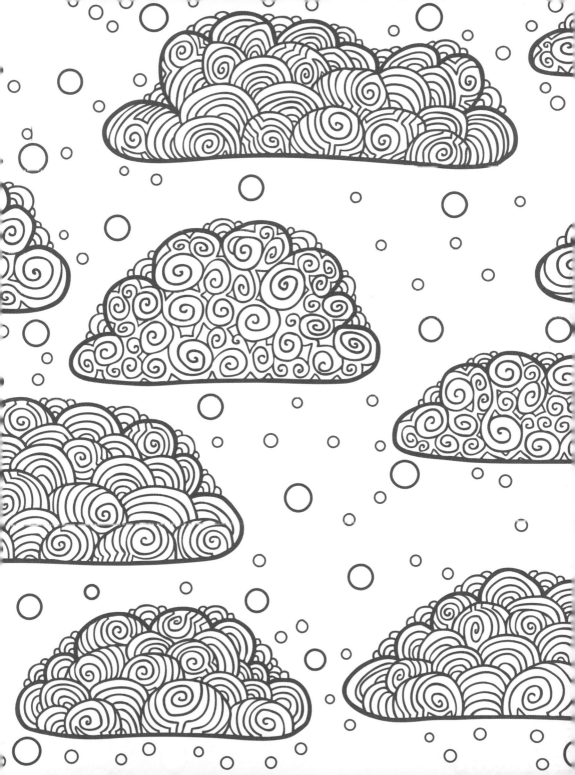

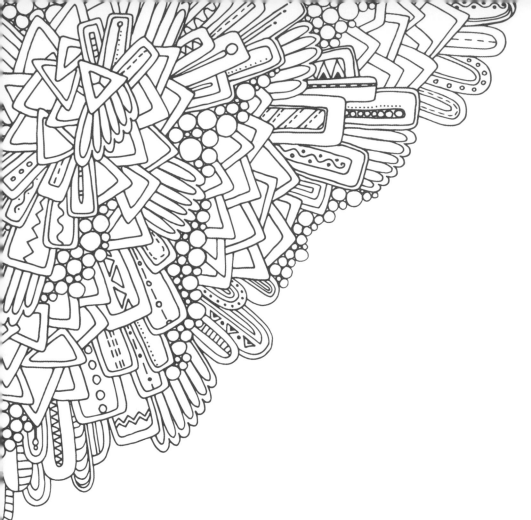

To be awake is to be alive.

Henry David Thoreau

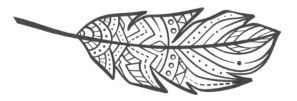

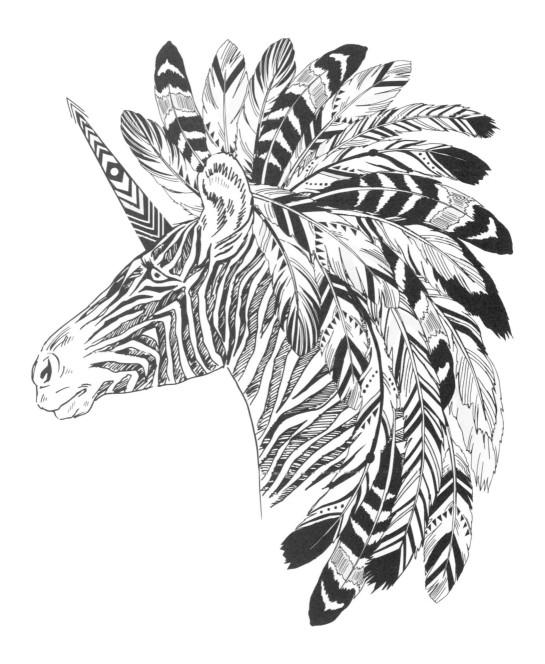

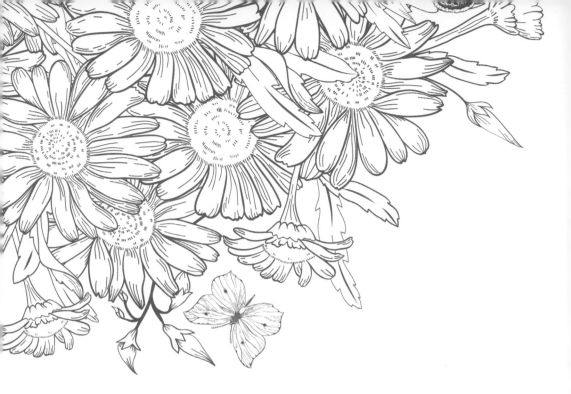

Drawing is a frame of mind,
A loving embrace, if you will.

Susan Avishai

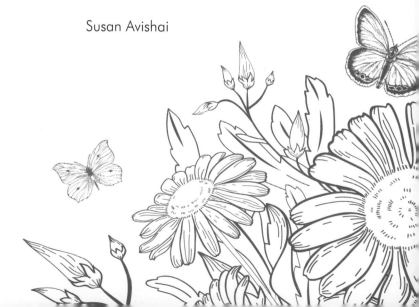

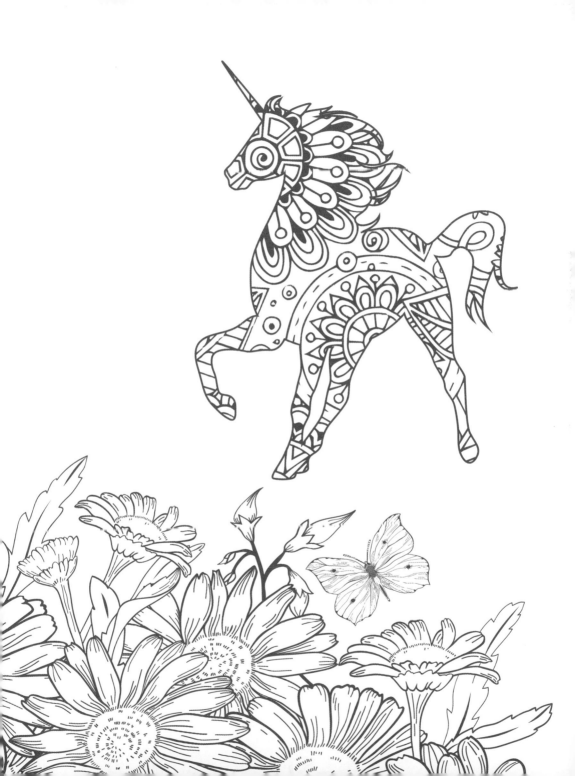

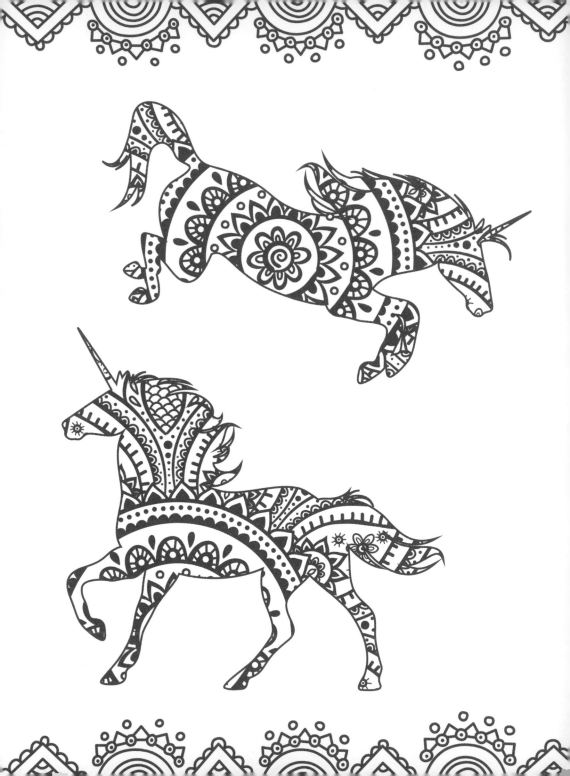

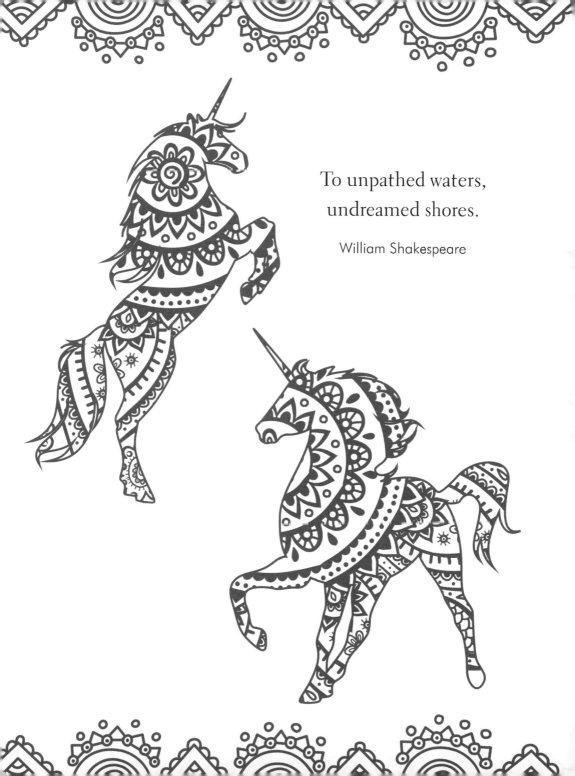

To unpathed waters,
undreamed shores.

William Shakespeare

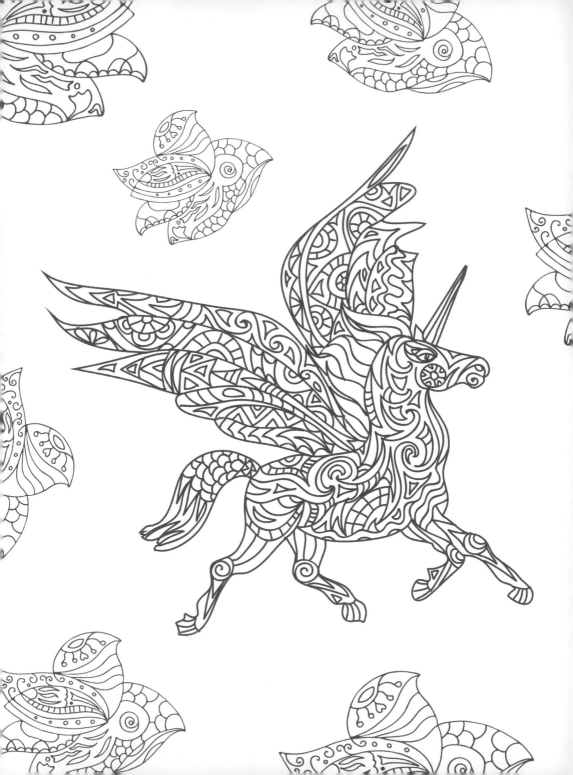

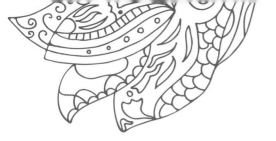
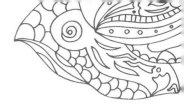
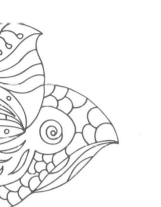
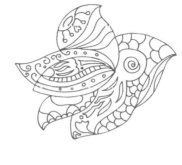
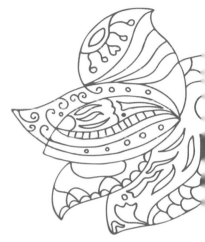
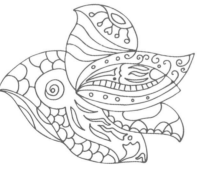
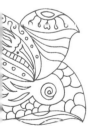
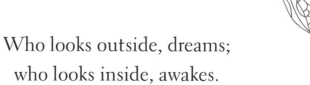

Who looks outside, dreams;
who looks inside, awakes.

Carl Jung

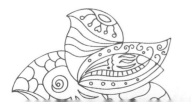
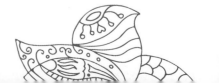

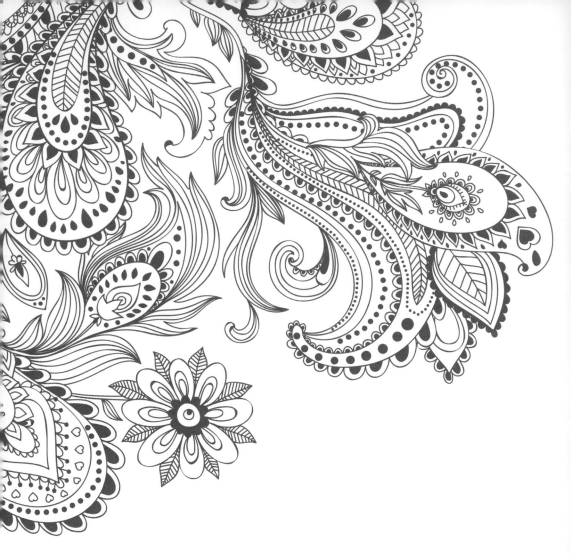

You are never too old to set another
goal or to dream a new dream.

C. S. Lewis

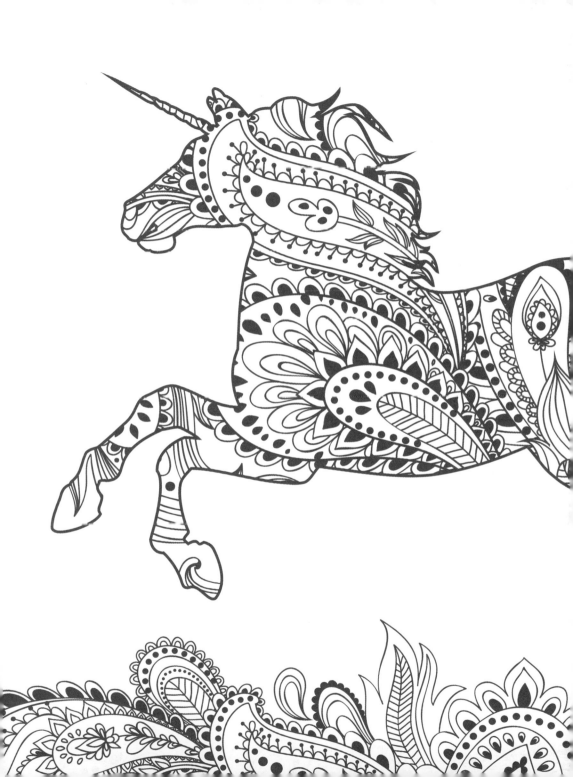

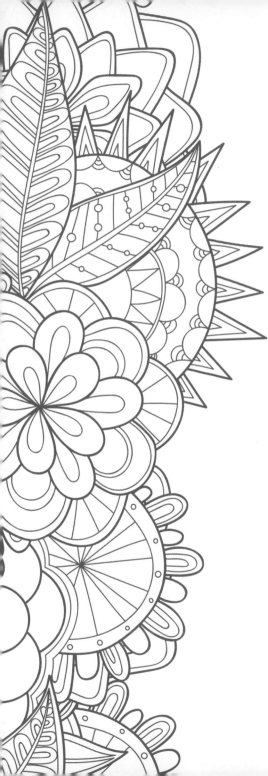

Imagination is more
important than knowledge.
For knowledge is limited,
whereas imagination
encircles the entire world.

Albert Einstein

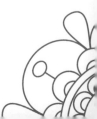

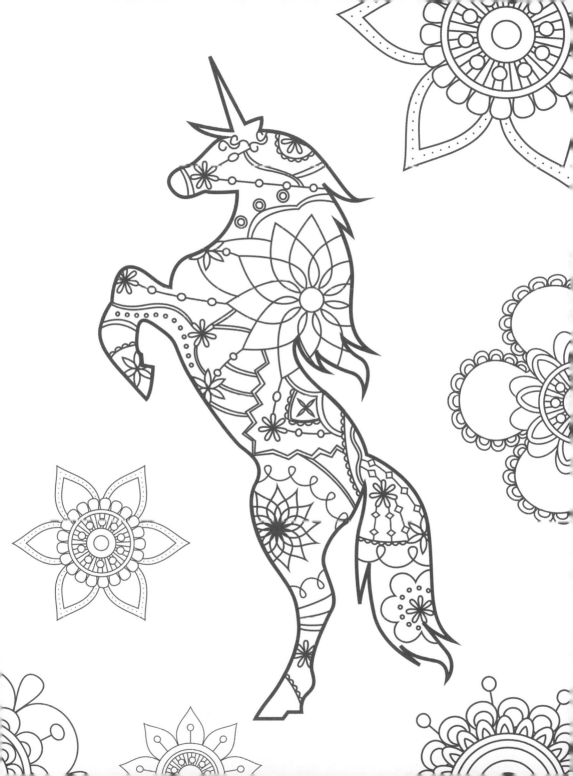

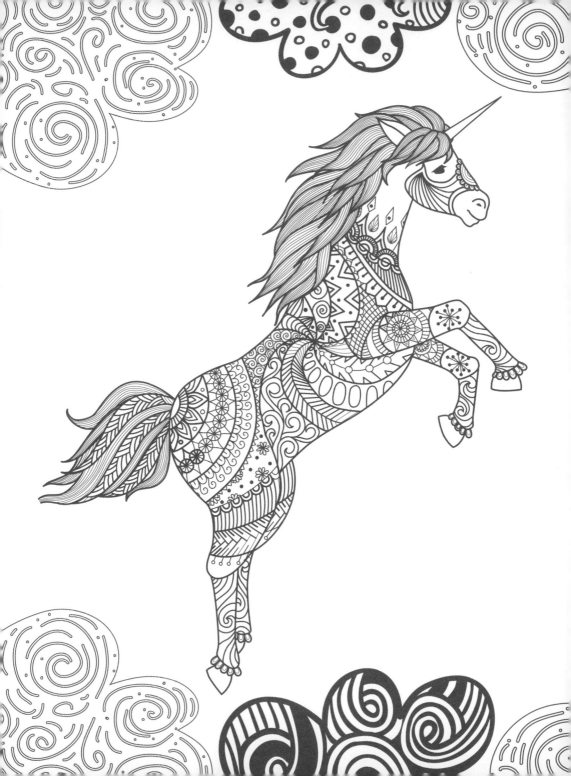

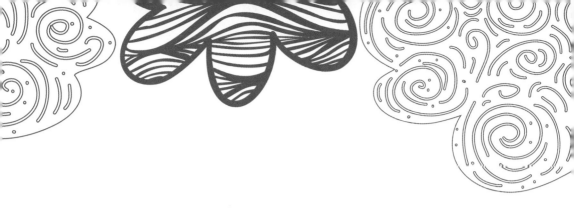

The world is but a canvas to our imagination.

Henry David Thoreau

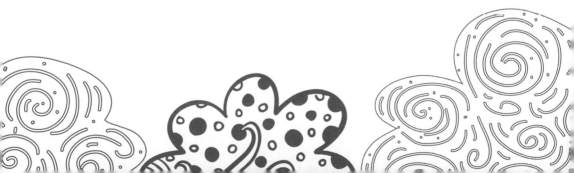

The purest and most thoughtful minds…

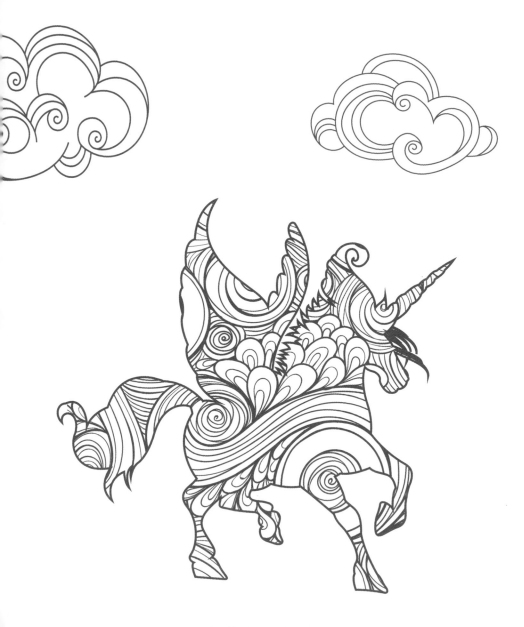

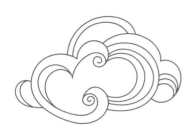

... are those which love colour the most.

John Ruskin

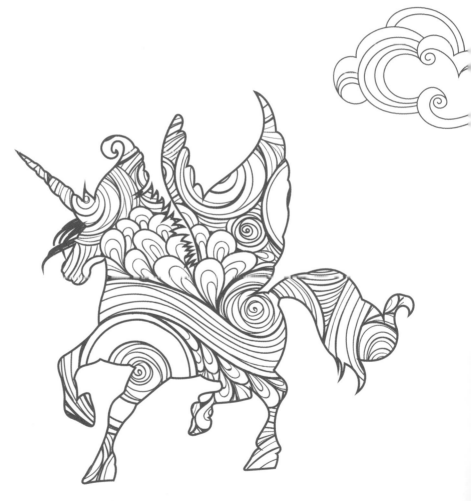

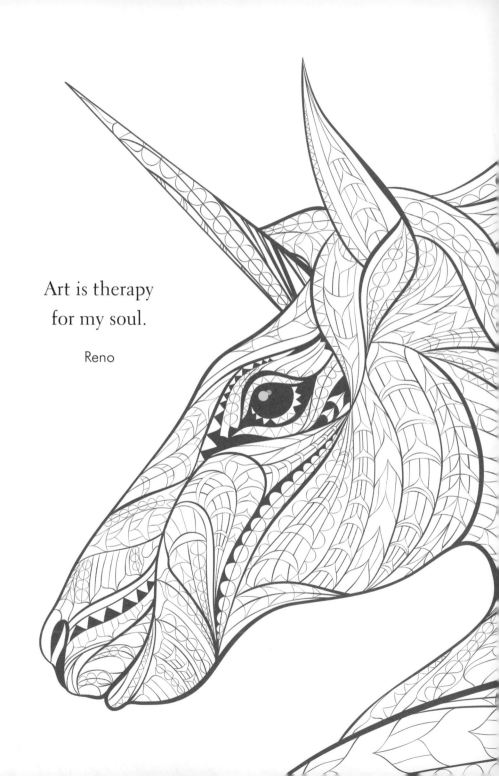

Art is therapy
for my soul.

Reno

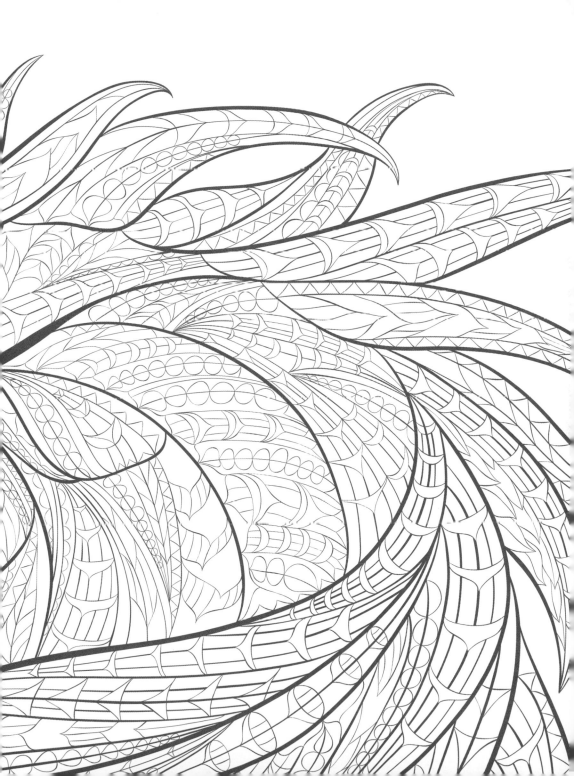

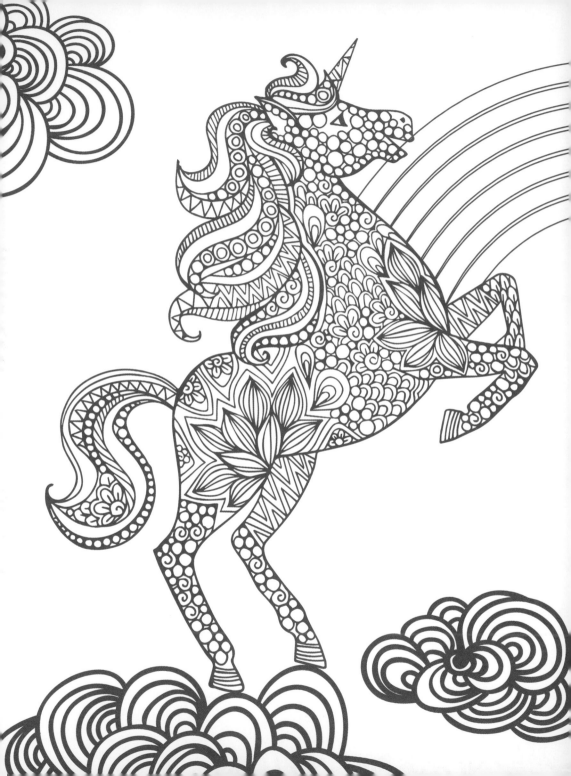

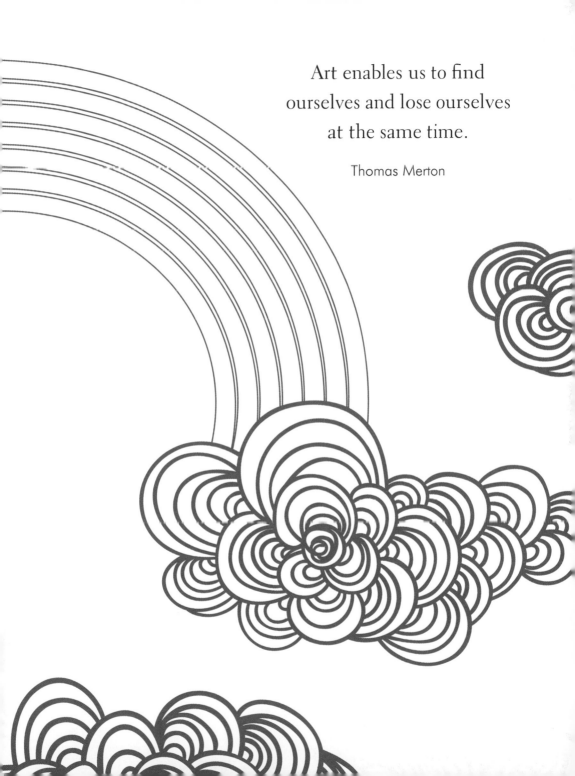

Art enables us to find
ourselves and lose ourselves
at the same time.

Thomas Merton

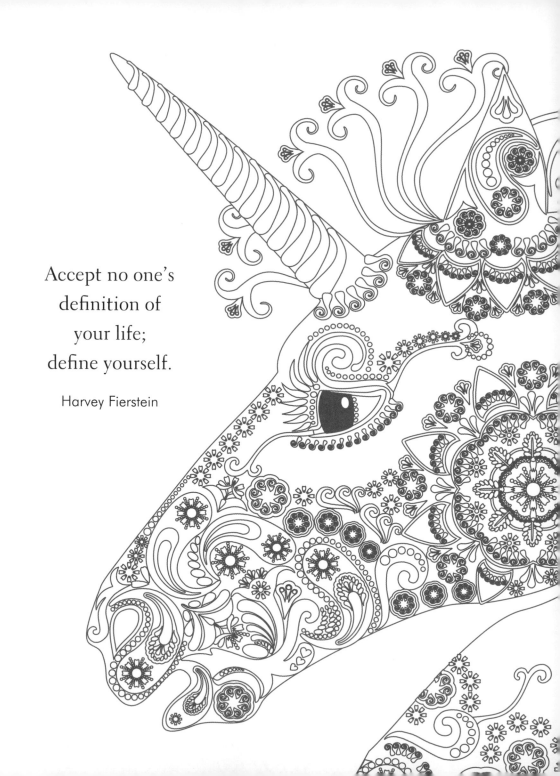

Accept no one's
definition of
your life;
define yourself.

Harvey Fierstein

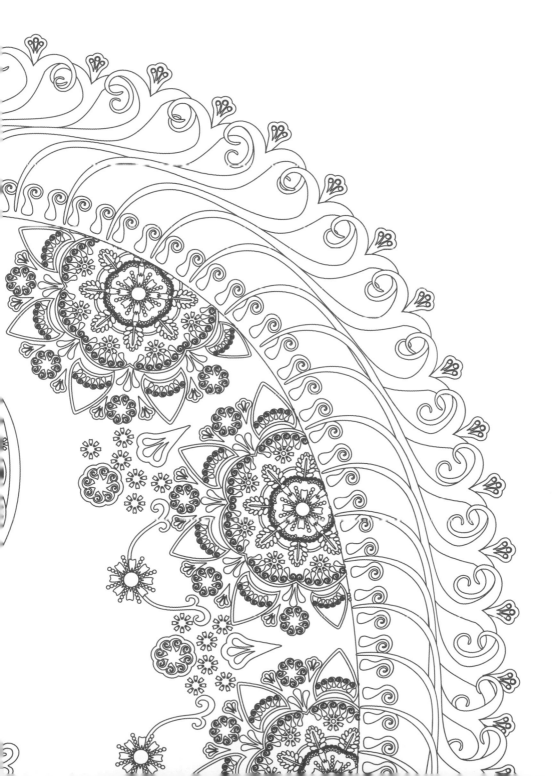

Put your ear down close to your soul
and listen hard.

Anne Sexton

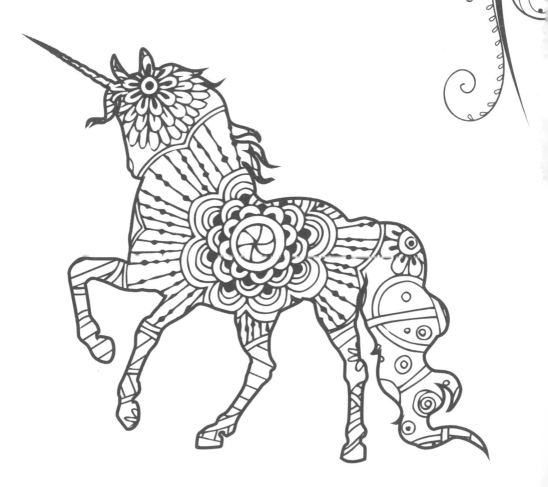

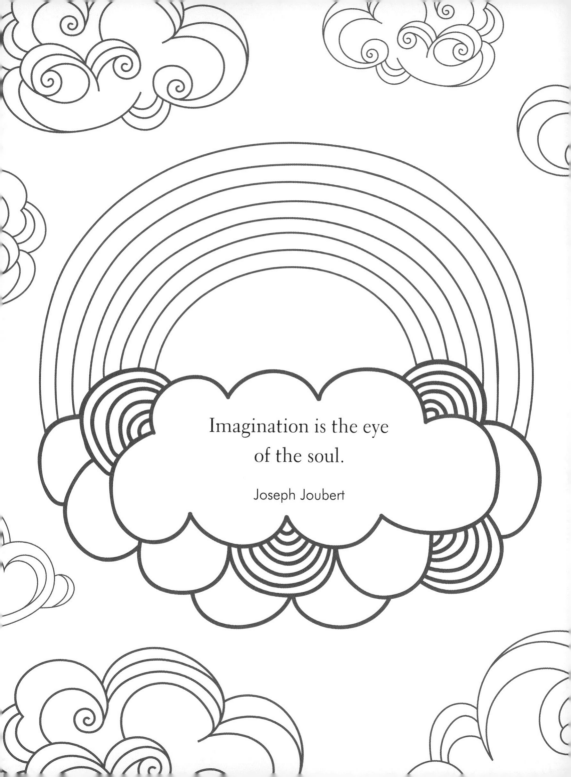

Imagination is the eye
of the soul.

Joseph Joubert

The pursuit, even of the best things,
ought to be calm and tranquil.

Cicero

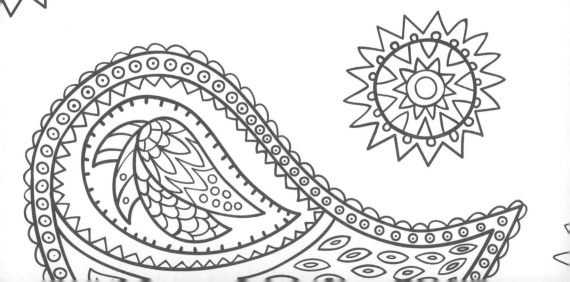

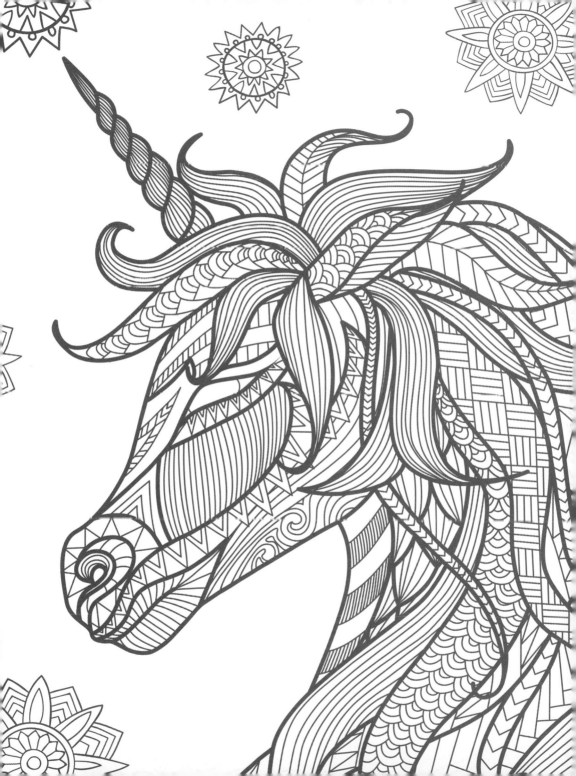

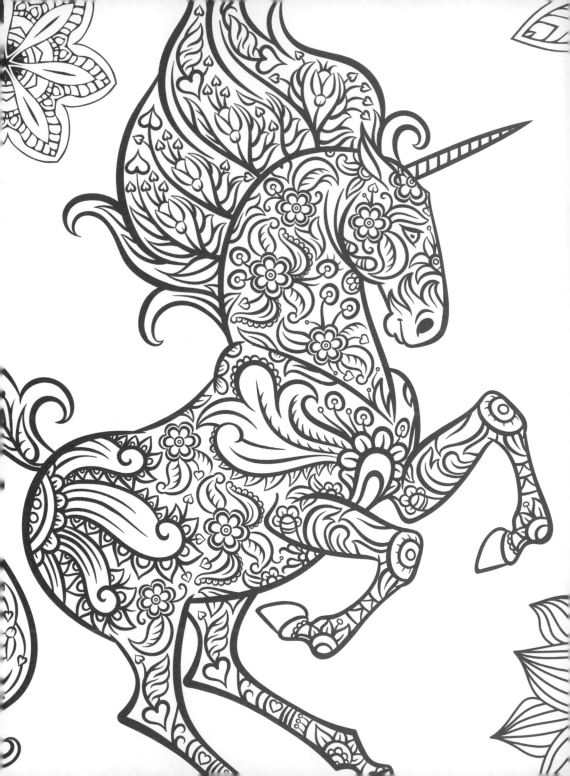

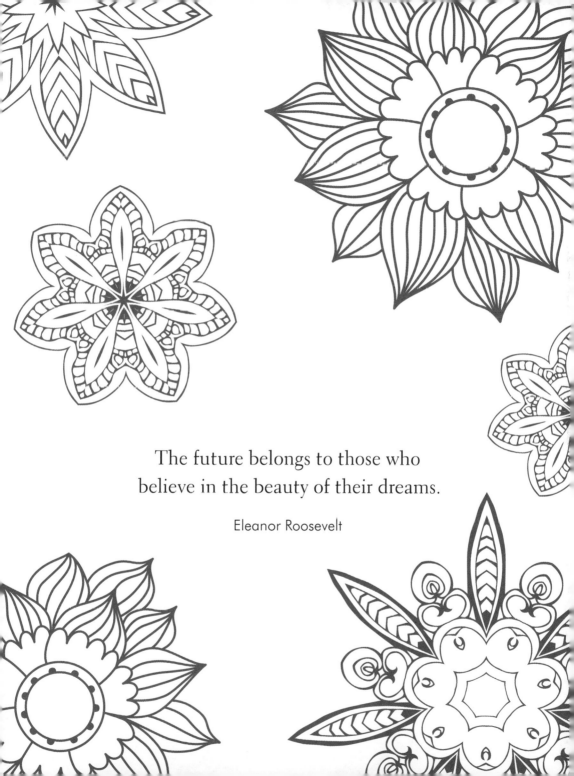

The future belongs to those who
believe in the beauty of their dreams.

Eleanor Roosevelt

Nobody can do everything, but
everyone can do something.

Anonymous

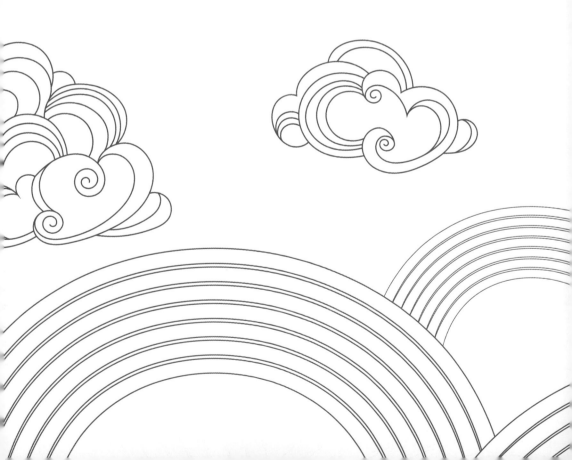

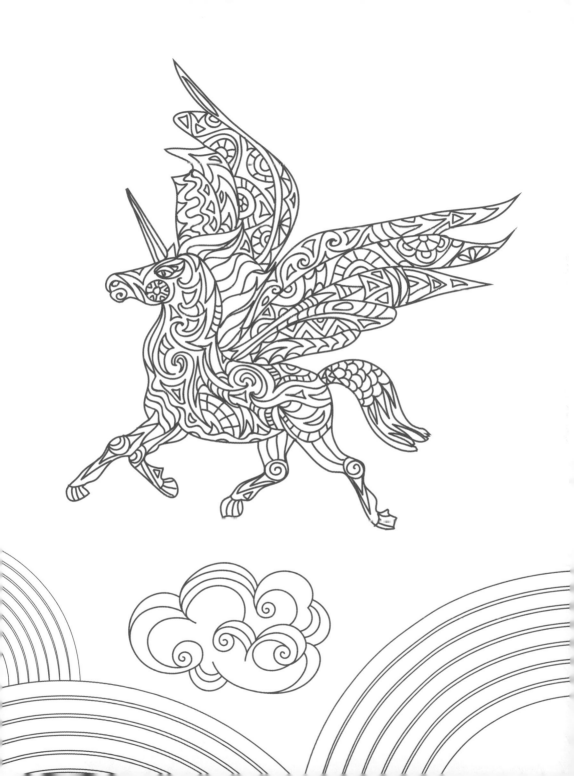

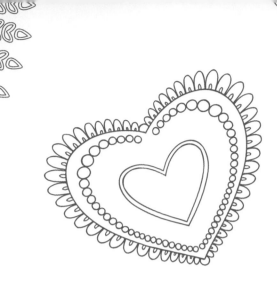

The world is but a canvas
to our imagination.

Henry David Thoreau

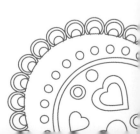

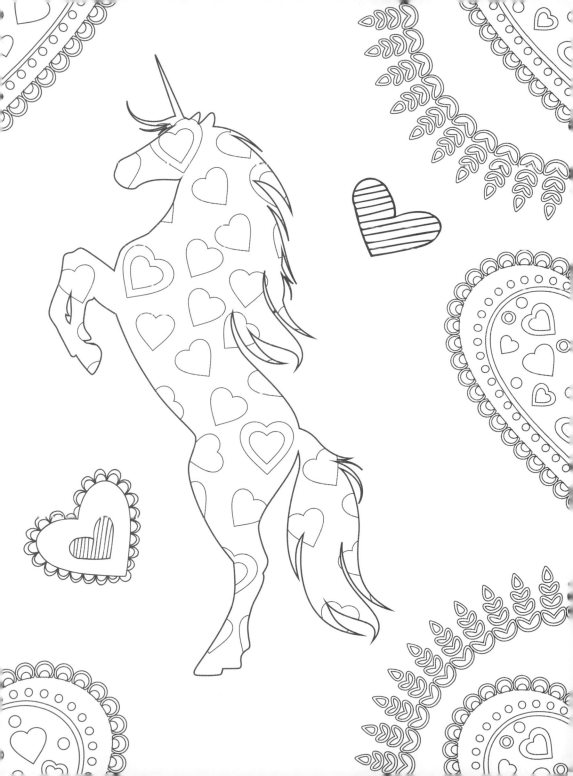

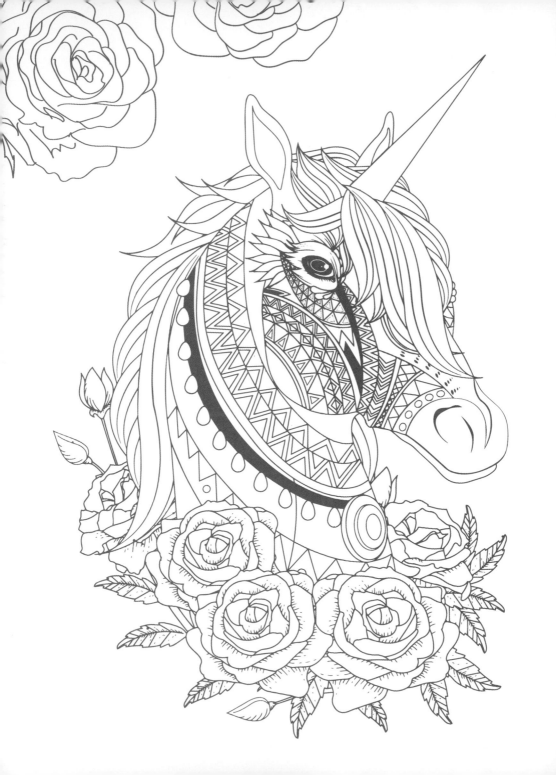

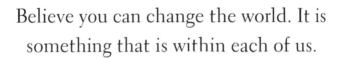

Believe you can change the world. It is
something that is within each of us.

Evan Tanner

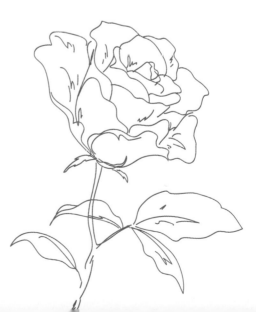

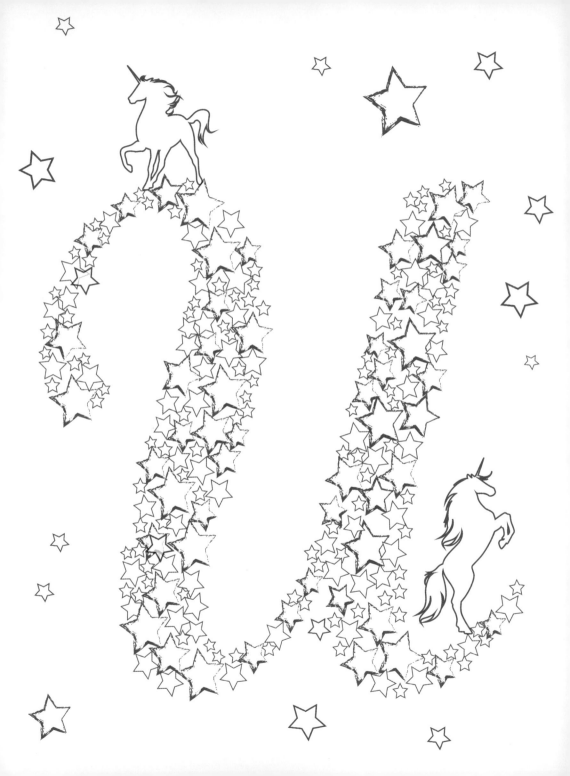

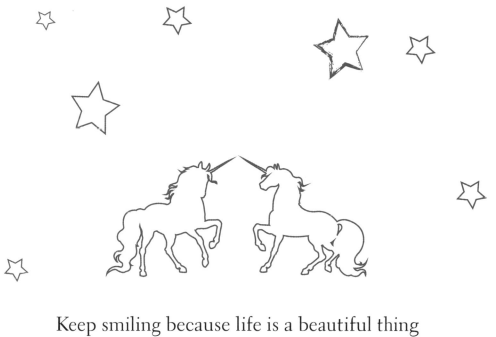

Keep smiling because life is a beautiful thing
and there's so much to smile about.

Marilyn Monroe

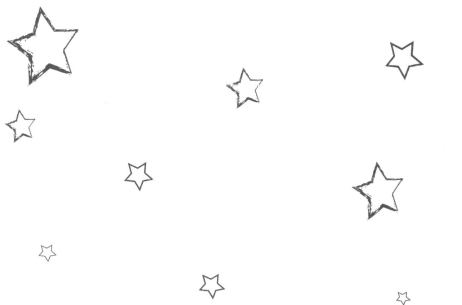

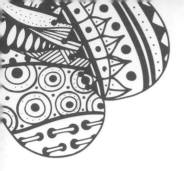
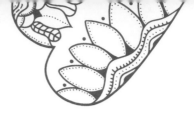

Get out of your head and into your
heart. Think less, feel more.

Osho

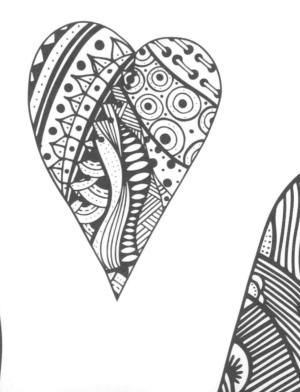

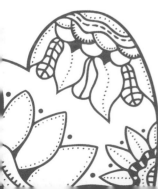

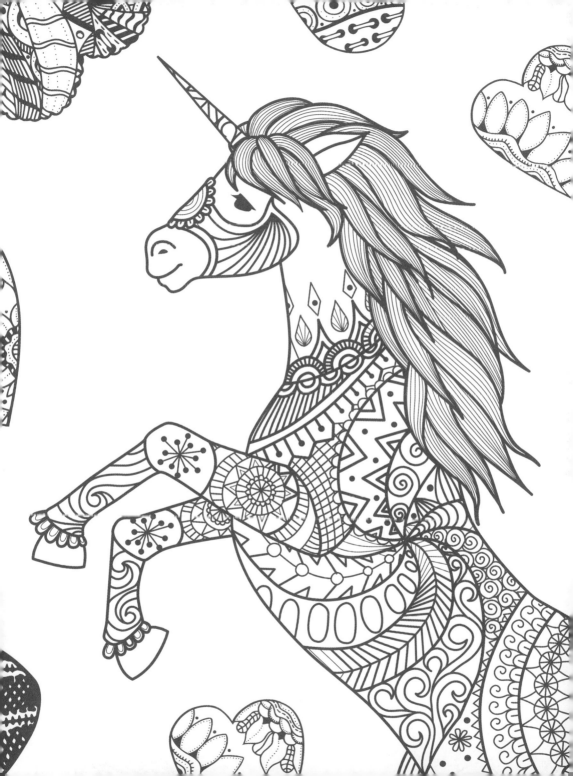

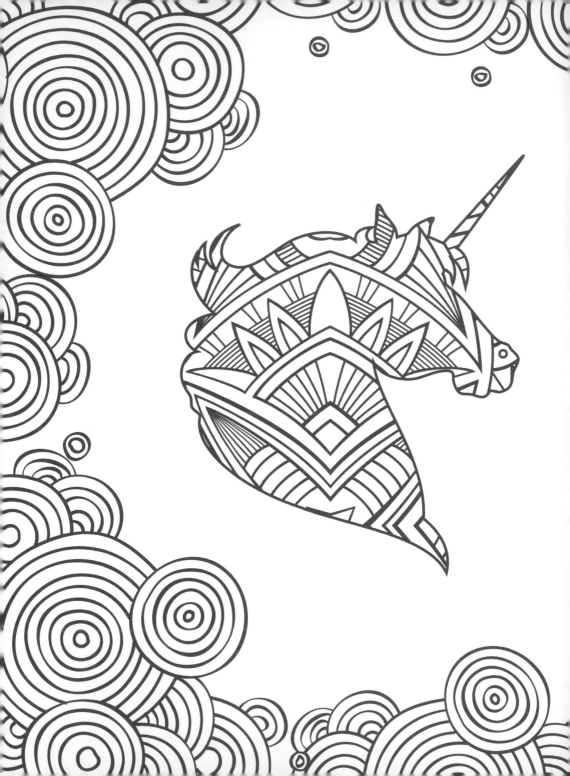

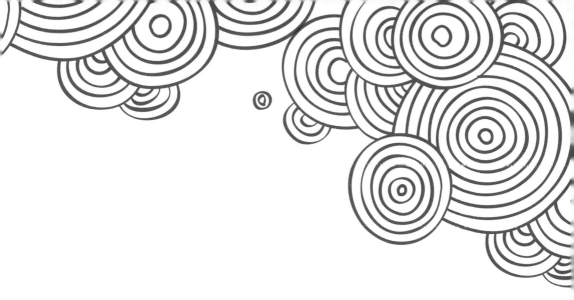

Each colour lives by its mysterious life.

Wassily Kandinsky

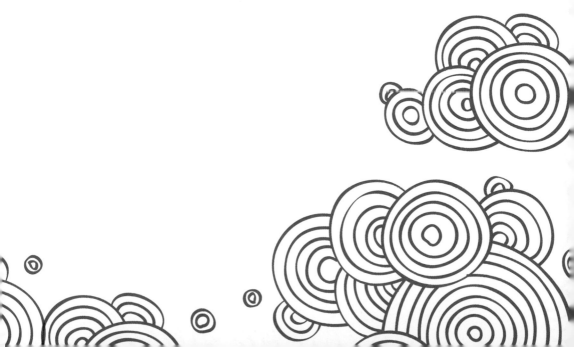

If you're interested in finding out
more about our products, find us on
Facebook at **HuckAndPucker** and
follow us on Twitter at @**HuckandPucker**.

www.huckandpucker.com

KEEP CALM AND COLOUR UNICORNS

Copyright © Huck & Pucker, 2016

Huck & Pucker is an imprint of Summersdale Publishers Ltd

Cover images © Marina Sterina / Bimbim / lenkis art / frescomovie / Olga Yatsenko / Elena Barenbaum
(Shutterstock)

Images © Shutterstock

Huck & Pucker
Huck Towers
46 West Street
Chichester
West Sussex
PO19 1RP
UK

www.huckandpucker.com

Printed and bound in the UK by Bell and Bain Ltd, Glasgow

ISBN: 978-1-909865-25-9